The Fat Loss Prescription:

The Fat Loss Prescription:

The Nine-Step Plan to Losing Weight and Keeping It Off

DR. SPENCER NADOLSKY

ISBN: 1518824226
ISBN 13: 9781518824227

This book is dedicated to my patients. If you don't give up on me, I will not give up on you.

Table of Contents

Acknowledgments

WANT TO THANK my mother, Martje, who always said I could be a writer; my dad, Karl, who taught me to live my life through science; my brother, Kasey, who is my greatest mentor; and my wife, Jenna, who has supported my dreams.

I also want to thank my mentors from the Obesity Society, American Board of Obesity Medicine, Obesity Medicine Association (formerly American Society of Bariatric Physicians), National Lipid Association, and my attending physicians from residency, who taught me to be the best doctor I can be.

Disclaimer

T HIS BOOK CONTAINS advice and information related to medicine and health care. It should not replace the advice of your physician. If you want to implement the information in this book, please consult with your physician first. The author disclaims liability for any medical outcomes that may occur as a result of applying the information contained in this book.

Introduction

Why I Wrote This Book, and Why You Should Read It

"YOU JUST NEED to have more willpower."

"You just need to eat less and move more."

"You have to try harder."

As a doctor, I hear stories from patients every day; they tell me how their doctor, trainer, friends, and family tell them that they are just not trying hard enough to lose weight and that they are "lazy." The ironic thing is that my patients *have* been trying for years. In fact, many of my patients lost over forty pounds multiple times—only to gain it back—before coming to me.

Do they really need to just "try harder," or is there something else going on?

Since medical school, I have attended one or two big obesity conferences per year, listening to the smartest obesity physicians and researchers speak about the latest research in medicine, nutrition, and exercise and methods for keeping weight off. The presenters are the leading researchers in the world. When you see a study in the news about obesity, chances are one of these researchers conducted it or runs the lab where it was done.

When you look at all the work these researchers have done, four rules for weight loss emerge:

1. In some cases, a medical cause such as a disease or drug may make it harder to lose weight.
2. Almost all diet and exercise plans work in the short term but fail in the long term.

3. The most important key to weight-loss success is sticking to a program.
4. When you figure out *your* key to adherence, you'll be able to lose weight and keep it off.

Virtually every clinician and researcher in the obesity and weight-loss field shares the views mentioned above, which are backed by the best scientific evidence.

So why are there thousands of fad diet books and programs that completely ignore what these researchers are saying? You have diets that suggest avoiding all grains, diets that allow eating only vegetables, diets that eliminate all sugar, very low-carb diets, very low-fat diets, Paleo diets, Mediterranean diets, diets that involve intermittent fasting, and dozens of other "special" methods for weight loss.

The reason is that people want easy answers. And the funny thing is that all of these diets work, for a while. But none of them have solved obesity, and most don't work all that well in the long term. People get bored, hungry, or frustrated by lack of results, and they quit.

There are proven solutions to obesity, and some people are talking about them. But most people still don't know what to do. I wrote this book because I wanted to make the best and latest research on weight loss available to people like you, who don't have time to read through the studies or talk to leading medical experts. This book will answer the questions that have been on your mind for years, like:

- What diet and exercise plan should I try?
- Do I need a weight-loss medicine?
- When is it time to think about getting surgery?
- Are there medical reasons I might not be losing weight?
- Are my medicines making me gain weight?

In the first chapter, you'll learn *why* it's so easy to gain weight—and so hard to lose it. In the second chapter, you'll learn about my nine-step plan for fat loss and how it encompasses the best ways of losing weight and keeping it off. When I say "best," I don't mean the fastest. The nine-step fat-loss program can cause rapid weight loss, but the main goal is *sustainable* weight loss. You'll learn how to make consistent lifestyle changes that allow you to lose weight and keep it off without feeling hungry or deprived all of the time.

You'll also learn about the conditions and medications that may be hindering your weight loss. If following the nine steps doesn't work for you, you'll learn about other weight-loss methods to consider, including medications and surgery. By the end of this book, you will know how to adhere to a diet-and-exercise plan for life. It doesn't matter how much fat you lose in a few months—what matters is how well you can maintain your new weight for years. That's the only way you'll be able to stay lean long term.

Throughout the book, you'll also learn what to discuss with your doctor. He or she will play an important role in guiding you through this process. If your doctor isn't able to help you, this book will show you how to find someone who can.

Finally, this book isn't about achieving a "perfect weight" or some sort of "ideal body." It's about empowering you to find what leading obesity specialists Arya Sharma and Yoni Freedhoff call your "best weight." Your best weight is the "sweet spot" where you're healthiest and happiest without having to be miserable following a rigid plan.

Part 1

The FLP Steps to Lasting Weight Loss

1

It's Not Your Fault: Why It's So Easy to Gain Weight (and So Hard to Lose It)

YOU'VE LOST WEIGHT in the past.

Maybe it was five pounds. Maybe it was twenty or even fifty. But the fact that you're reading this book means you probably didn't keep it off.

That's nothing to be ashamed of. Most people can't lose weight and keep it off. The problem is that most of us don't reflect on *why* this is true.

If you've failed to maintain a healthy weight, it's easy to beat yourself up. You may think any of the following:

"I must have bad genetics. I guess I'm stuck like this."
"I'm just weak—I don't have the willpower to make this work."
"I must have a slow metabolism."

If you want to maintain a healthy weight, however, beating yourself up doesn't work. You have to look deeper into why you weren't able to stay lean in the past. Then we can work together to fix those issues.

There are many factors working against maintaining a healthy body weight. Let's look at some of the major ones.

Your Genes and Your Environment Are Working against You

Thirty-two-year-old Becky had been told by everyone from family to friends to co-workers that she just needed to "eat less" to lose weight. Becky was a busy mom with a demanding position as a sales manager who excelled in every other area of her life. While she was always trying to diet, Becky often felt hungry and had cravings for junk food. Her family and friends considered her lazy because she couldn't lose weight. They made it even harder for her by constantly eating high-calorie junk food around her. They were basically telling her that she needed to work harder to lose weight while sabotaging her efforts to eat less. How nice.

Unfortunately, Becky's story is common. Your environment—the people, places, things, and foods you surround yourself with—has a huge impact on your ability to lose weight. You've probably read articles about how our modern environment makes it easy to gain weight. We have convenience stores everywhere. Soda, french fries, and candy are cheaper than fresh fruit and vegetables. Most jobs don't require you to get out of your chair. Our modern comforts, like television and pre-packaged meals, also make it easy to gain weight.

You may have also read about how some people have "fat" genes and others have "skinny" ones. You've heard that some people are destined to be overweight while others are destined to be thin, regardless of how they eat.

So which is it that determines body weight—environment or genetics?

Both.

Let's look at environment first. Some foods are "hyperpalatable," meaning they have a combination of ingredients that overrides our body's normal satiety cues. These foods are generally high in refined carbohydrates and fat, like potato chips and candy. Basically these foods give us a bunch of calories without filling us up—and leave us wanting more and more. If you eat these foods, you're more likely to gain weight.

It's not only the food you eat that can affect you—certain viruses, such as adeno-virus-36, a common cold virus, may cause you to gain weight. That virus only affects about 30 percent of people with obesity, but it's still one more unexpected way your environment is working against you.

Many other environmental factors affect our weight as well, such as money, time, where we live, etc. Some of these are in our control, and some aren't. We just have to learn how to best deal with our environment, which is what we will discuss in this book.

Unfortunately, your genes do play a role in your weight as well. I try not to dwell on this too much with patients because there is nothing you can do about it. However, while your genes have a large impact on your ability to lose weight, your *epigenetics* may be even more important. Epigenetics is the study of how your environment influences the expression of different genes. Your genes work like an old-fashioned telephone switchboard. When you, the operator, do certain behaviors, you flip some genes "on" and others "off." Those genes send signals to other parts of your body, which influence your health and body composition.

If you're sedentary and sit around a lot, inactivity turns off the genes that help protect you against heart disease. When you start a smart exercise program, however, those genes are turned on and your risk of heart disease decreases.

Then there is metabolic programming. If your mother was overweight, sedentary, and ate a poor diet, your chances of gaining fat increase. Your mother's decisions even while you were in the womb have a direct impact on your risk of obesity. You're stuck with the consequences of your mother's behavior. It's not fair, but that's how it is.

None of this is meant for you to lose hope. I only mean to show that your current weight right now is not all your fault.

When I met Becky, I explained that her hunger and cravings weren't a result of lack of willpower or discipline. And she clearly wasn't lazy—she worked her tail off in every other aspect of her life. But she was making her cravings worse by what she was eating—junk food that tasted good but never satisfied her. This made sense to her.

Together Becky and I built a diet-and-exercise plan and support system. We worked together to change her environment so she could stick to the plan long term. She lost fifty pounds in nine months and has kept it off.

Becky had many things working against her—her family, her environment, her job—but by changing her habits, she was able to change her body. You may not always be able to control your environment, and you can't control your genes, but you can control your habits.

Your Habits May Be Working against You

Think about how you've tried to lose weight before. At some point, you probably tried to follow a rigid diet and exercise plan like the Atkins diet or P90X. And what happened? You may have felt great at first, but after a few weeks, you got bored and quit—or you just hated it after a while.

You may also have tried to take a more moderate approach. You served yourself smaller portions and walked every day. You lost even more weight that time, but eventually, your weight stalled and then crept back up.

So what's the problem?

You didn't change your habits.

Most of your daily actions are habits. You might think things like picking broccoli over cake or walking instead of watching TV are conscious choices, but they often aren't. Studies indicate that around 40 percent of your daily behaviors are subconscious habits instead of logical choices.

You've probably experienced this yourself. You work out for a few weeks, but over time you find yourself falling back into watching TV and surfing the Internet at night instead.

Over the past two decades, scientists have gained a much better understanding of how habits form and how we can change them. A habit is basically an unconscious "script" that's encoded into your memory and helps your brain work more efficiently.

Your brain is much better at focusing on one thing at a time. When you learn a new task, your brain is looking for ways to save energy. It wants to master the new task as fast as possible so it can do it better next time. This is true for every behavior you do on a regular basis.

When you first learned to drive, your brain was working overtime trying to master the new skill. Now you probably don't even think about how much pressure you put on the gas pedal or how you move the steering wheel—it happens automatically. That's a habit.

The more you practice a habit, the more ingrained it becomes. Driving is now almost effortless for you. Habits also remain encoded in your brain for years. If you started driving again after five years of not driving, you'd still be decent. Maybe a little rusty at first, but not bad. Your driving habits are still there; they just need a little practice. The same thing happens when you choose what to buy at the grocery store or decide whether to watch TV or go for a walk after work.

If you've been eating junk food for years, it will take time to "unlearn" those habits and form new ones. The same is true if you've been sitting on a couch or behind a computer for years instead of exercising.

There is good news when it comes to habits—*you can create healthy habits* just as easily as you can create unhealthy ones. With practice, it will actually be easier to work out than to sit on the couch after work. It will feel weird to pick macaroni and cheese instead of a salad at lunch.

It takes time and practice, and you'll learn how to change those habits for the better later in the book. For now, just remember that most of your choices are dictated by habits and that habits take time to change.

Deon's Story: Turn a Bad Habit into a Good One

Deon, forty-two, worked all day as a security guard and then came home to dinner with his wife and kids. He would crack open a soda or two and sit and watch the news until bedtime. Unfortunately, his waistline and blood pressure didn't appreciate this. He was 253 pounds with a forty-three-inch waist and a blood pressure of 145/92. He came to me for advice.

After going over Deon's diet and exercise history, it seemed the best thing he could do was change his postdinner ritual. He lived in a neighborhood where it was easy to walk, so I asked if he was willing to go for a walk with his wife each night after dinner. His wife, who was with him, was excited at the idea, and Deon agreed to it.

After focusing on this habit every day for two months, Deon had lost nine pounds. This may not seem like much, but it gave him the jump-start he needed to start a more formal exercise plan, similar to the one in this book. His blood pressure is now normal (under 120/80), he's lost five inches off his waist, and he no longer needs blood pressure medication. And his relationship with his wife is better than ever!

"Diets" Don't Work

If you've been trying to lose weight for a while, you've probably researched many different approaches. You've read at least ten different diet books. You read diet blogs. You get advice from friends and family. It seems like the only thing these diets agree on is that vegetables are good for you. The rest of their advice seems horribly contradictory:

"Carbs are bad."
"Carbs are good."

"Fat is bad."

"Fat is good."

"Fruit makes you fat."

"Animal meat gives you cancer."

"Fiber is bad for you."

"Grapefruit detoxes your body."

"Putting butter in your coffee burns belly fat."

This advice may be overwhelming, but you're sure that the only way to lose weight is to opt for the latest plan. So you give a diet (or probably more than one) an honest shot, but after a few weeks, you stop seeing results, or you get sick of them. Here's why.

For the past hundred years, every high-quality study has shown that if you want to lose fat, you have to eat fewer calories than you burn. Most fad diets work because they trick you into eating fewer calories. It's that simple.

Keep in mind that there's nothing stopping people from making things up ("I ate whatever I wanted and still lost weight!") to impress or mislead you, especially when they have something to sell.

So don't fall into the trap of believing that a fad diet is the answer to your weight-loss prayers. Fad diets don't work in the long term unless you stick with them forever (which is nearly impossible), and they don't work for the reasons people claim.

I caution patients against falling for fad diets; instead, I help people take a more flexible approach to dieting so they don't feel confined to a rigid eating pattern. You'll learn about those simple eating steps in the next chapter. For now, all I want you to know is that yes, there are factors working against your goal of losing weight and keeping it off. But you can accomplish your goal.

Sandra's Story: Hooked on the Latest Diet

Sandra is a fifty-year-old who *loved* to try new diets. She was always coming in and asking me about the new diet craze that her friends were trying or that she saw on the news. Every diet worked for her—at first. She would lose about thirty pounds and then gain it back when she stopped following whatever diet she was trying and returned to her old habits.

It wasn't the grains, the fructose, or the fat—it was her inability to stick to the plan that made it hard to keep the weight off. I had her start by changing one small habit at a time, like eating protein at every meal and walking after every meal. She worked with me and one of my coaches daily until she mastered each habit. She has currently lost a total of forty-four pounds and has kept it off for over two years. She doesn't yo-yo diet anymore, and she has no problem sticking to the diet because her habits are so well ingrained.

Short on Motivation?

If you're concerned about the factors working against you to lose weight, don't give up yet. Having personally worked with hundreds of patients who have overcome these factors and lost weight for good, I've found that they share similar reasons for changing their habits. Consider these powerful motivators:

You'll live longer and stay healthier. This is the number one reason to lose weight. You're less likely to get a number of diseases if you're leaner, and your life expectancy will increase too.

If your doctor has told you that you're overweight or obese, chances are that losing fat will improve your life. Studies have repeatedly shown that losing weight causes a massive improvement in blood lipids, blood pressure, blood vessel health, and insulin sensitivity. Weight loss also reduces the severity of sleep disorders like sleep apnea, which can have a negative impact on every other part of your life.

The bottom line is that by losing weight, you'll spend less time in doctors' offices and hospitals—and more time doing things you enjoy.

You'll feel better on a day-to-day basis. Imagine that you could jump off the couch and go outside to play with your dog. Imagine that you could run up the stairs without getting winded. Imagine that you could go hiking on a whim with a friend.

When you're leaner, you're able to do these things and enjoy life more. Simple things like walking up a flight of stairs won't be so frustrating. Finding clothes that fit won't be so hard. Most of all, improving your weight gives you a boost in confidence. You know you're taking care of yourself, which improves your outlook and attitude throughout the day.

You don't have to lose much weight to get benefits. If you're worried that losing weight will be too difficult, keep in mind that it can be hardest at the beginning, when you're initially changing your habits. After a few weeks, however, changing your habits starts to get easier and easier. In most cases, you'll see massive results with only a few changes to your daily routine.

The awesome thing is that you don't need to lose much weight to see significant benefits. Studies have shown that losing as little as 5 percent of your starting weight can drastically lower your risk of heart disease, stroke, and diabetes. I've had many patients who weighed two hundred to three hundred pounds no longer need medication for high blood pressure and high blood sugars after losing only ten or fifteen pounds.

The bottom line is that you can change. I've worked with hundreds of people who felt hopeless at first yet completely changed their lives with a few simple habits. These people aren't special. They're not all that different from you. They lost weight for good, and you can too.

As you can see, it's not really your fault if you've gained weight and haven't been able to lose it. Many factors are working against you. We'll talk about overcoming those factors and changing your bad habits into healthier ones in the next chapter.

2

The Fat Loss Prescription: The Nine-Step Plan to Losing Weight and Keeping It Off

Now you know the primary reasons why it's so hard to lose weight and keep it off—and why fad diets don't work in the long run. What does? Small, doable changes to the way you're living now. My Fat Loss Prescription (FLP) includes nine simple steps in three areas: how you eat, how you move, and how you live.

I promise it's not as hard or complicated as you might think. I've used these same methods with hundreds of patients who didn't think they could lose weight, and they did. What's more, 90 percent of them have kept off the weight for years.

The nine-step fat loss prescription is comprised of the following:

How You Eat

FLP Step #1: Your diet should help you eat fewer calories than you burn and help you eat enough protein.

FLP Step #2: Your diet should consist of mostly nutrient-rich foods.

FLP Step #3: Your diet must be enjoyable for the long term.

How You Move

FLP Step #4: Exercise regularly.

FLP Step #5: Lift weights *and* do aerobic exercise.

FLP Step #6: Make movement a part of your daily routine.

How You Live
FLP Step #7: Get more, and better quality, sleep.
FLP Step #8: Seek out a weight-loss support group.
FLP Step #9: Find ways to handle emotions that don't involve food.

In this chapter, we'll focus on the three dietary steps, as I've found these are the biggest barriers to weight loss. In later chapters, we'll address how you move and how you live.

FLP #1: Your diet should help you eat fewer calories than you burn and help you eat enough protein.

First, keep in mind that there's no such thing as the "perfect" diet. But if you want to lose weight, you need to change how you're eating today. How much of a change you need to make depends on the quality (and quantity) of your diet. Some people have to make significant changes to their diet to see results, like drastically reducing how much junk food they eat or learning how to cook. Others may only need to make a few small tweaks, like cutting out sodas, to lose a significant amount of weight.

Regardless, the goal of the first step is to create a "calorie deficit." By consuming fewer calories than your body burns, you will lose weight. The best way to create a calorie deficit is with a sustainable diet. Exercise is important too, but it's almost never enough by itself to cause significant weight loss. To sustain a calorie deficit, you'll need to follow a diet that makes it easy to keep your calories low without getting too hungry.

The simplest, most effective way to do this is by following these strategies:

1. Get most of your calories from high-quality whole foods. Limit junk food, processed food, and high-fat, high-sugar fast food.
2. Use mindful eating techniques to control your portions by focusing on the food you're eating and checking in with your body to determine whether you're hungry or full. Make eating a stand-alone activity; in other words, don't eat while you're reading, watching TV, working, or driving—you'll eat more without realizing it and won't feel as satisfied.

3. Use smaller containers and serving dishes (like a salad plate instead of a dinner plate) so that your portions seem larger than they are.
4. Drink calorie-free beverages like water, coffee, and tea instead of soda, juice, and sports drinks. (Diet sodas and artificially sweetened drinks are better than regular sugary drinks.) If you must have alcohol, limit consumption to one or two drinks per day at most. Choose lower-calorie drinks like vodka, rum, gin, whiskey, or light beer; avoid alcoholic beverages with lots of added sugar.
5. Track your food intake, if necessary. (We'll cover diet tracking later in this section.)

Your diet is not just about calories—it should also help you eat enough protein.

One of the most common mistakes people make when trying to lose weight is that they fail to eat enough protein. Protein is extremely important for losing weight for three primary reasons:

- Protein keeps you feeling full and decreases your urge to eat more so than fat or carbs do.
- Protein helps you preserve muscle mass as you lose weight, which improves your body composition (your proportion of muscle to fat), and helps you lose a higher percentage of fat.
- Protein requires slightly more calories to digest than fat or carbs do.

A simple way to get enough protein for the day is to make sure you consume protein at every meal. A good rule of thumb is to aim for thirty to fifty grams of protein at each meal, assuming you're eating three meals per day along with one high-protein snack. Protein shakes work well as meal replacements.

FLP #2: Your diet should consist of mostly nutrient-rich whole foods.

In most cases, this means a wide variety of fresh fruits, vegetables, legumes, nuts and healthy oils, low-fat dairy, and lean meats.

A simple rule of thumb for meals is that one-half to three-quarters of your plate should contain different kinds of vegetables, fruits and/or legumes, and the remainder should be some kind of lean protein. Healthy fats like olive oil and nuts can be included as well. You can also throw some whole grains or starches on your plate, such as whole-wheat bread, potatoes, rice, and pasta, but the focus should be on vegetables, fruit, and legumes, as these are the lowest calorie foods that will fill you up.

It's okay to have dessert and less-healthy foods (e.g., chips) every now and then, but you should have these foods only occasionally—not every day. You'll learn more about reasonable indulgences in a moment.

You don't need to follow an exact list of foods, and your healthy diet might look very different from someone else's. I do, however, give patients a basic list of healthy foods to base their diet on:

Vegetables (Most of your diet should be vegetables, fruit, and legumes.)
Green leafy veggies (kale, spinach, etc.), broccoli, cauliflower, zucchini, onions, peppers, etc.

Fruit (Aim for at least one to two servings a day as a good starting place.)
Berries (blueberries, strawberries, etc.), melon, apples, oranges, bananas, avocados, etc.

Meat/Fish/Seafood (Have one to two servings of protein per meal.)
Lean beef (such as sirloin, round, and strip steak that is 93 percent lean or higher); chicken, turkey, or seafood (fish, shrimp, crab, etc.).

Dairy/Eggs (These can be part of the one to two servings of protein per meal.)
Eggs (whole and whites), cottage cheese, plain yogurt (Greek, regular, kefir, etc.), low-fat cheeses, regular-fat cheeses in moderation, and whey-based and other dairy-based protein powders.

Legumes (Most of your diet should be vegetables, fruit, and legumes.)
Beans (black, pinto, kidney, garbonzo etc.), lentils, etc.

Nuts/Oils (Limit to one or two servings per meal; one serving is about the size of your thumb.)
Walnuts, almonds, pistachios, cashews, pecans, peanuts (technically legumes but they contain healthy fat), olive oil, macadamia oil, almond oil, and most other plant-based oils.

Whole grains and potatoes (Serving size depends on your preferences and needs, which you'll learn about later.)

Oats, boiled or baked potatoes (sweet or white/yellow), brown rice, quinoa, etc.

Potatoes: Vegetable or Whole Grain?

Technically, potatoes are vegetables, but I list them here with the whole grains because they are higher in carbohydrates and calories than most other veggies. If you boil them or bake them, their nutritional value is very good. They can fill you up without a lot of calories. It's the frying (think potato chips and french fries) that makes them less healthy. I have my patients continue to eat potatoes as long as they don't fry them or soak them with butter and sour cream.

FLP Step #3: Your diet must be enjoyable for the long term.

It doesn't matter how "scientific" or "effective" your diet looks on paper if you can't stick to it. The single biggest mistake people make when trying to lose weight is following a diet they don't enjoy.

Most people think that dieting should feel hard, and that the harder the diet, the better it works. That's not true. Sure, dieting can be tough at times, but overall it should be enjoyable. Otherwise you'll never be able to stick to it. Here are some of the most effective strategies for creating a diet that you can enjoy for the long term.

Eat foods that you enjoy.

Eat a variety of fruits, vegetables, lean meats, seafood, low-fat dairy, nuts, seeds, and starches. As long as you're getting most of your calories from those foods, you can eat what you want. Don't feel like you have to eat chicken and broccoli because *Men's Health* said so. Quantity matters as well, which we will discuss in a moment.

Eat protein and produce at every meal.

This is one of the easiest and most effective methods for eating a healthy diet. Include a source of protein and some vegetables, fruit, or legumes at each meal. This helps you get enough protein throughout the day, stay full between meals, and get enough quality nutrition. Here are some simple targets for portion sizes:

- A palm-sized portion of lean meat like chicken, fish, or steak.
- A fist-sized portion of lean dairy like low-fat yogurt or milk.
- A scoop or two of protein powder.
- A fist-sized portion of legumes like chickpeas.
- Two fist-sized servings of fruit or vegetables.

What about bread and pasta? You can still have them, but focus on the above first. These foods will fill you up with fewer calories. In fact, one of the habits I help my patients develop is doubling their vegetables and cutting their starches (like pasta and potatoes) in half. For example, if you are used to taking two scoops of rice or pasta at dinner and one scoop of vegetables, switch to one scoop of rice or pasta and two scoops of vegetables. Easy.

If you do that at every meal, I promise you will see results.

Choosing the Best Whole Grains

Whole grains have gotten a lot of bad press recently. My problem with eating whole grains stems from the fact that many boxed sugary cereals and other junk claim they are full of whole grains—yet they're far from healthy. This is ridiculous. Skip the cereals and stick with "pure" whole grains like plain oats. For breakfast, have a serving of plain oatmeal with some protein powder and one or two servings of fruit and nuts. This is an awesome, healthy meal that will keep you full for hours.

Putting the Plan into Practice: A Day's Worth of Healthy Meals

I've given you the template for healthy meals. Now here are some examples of meals I eat and suggest my patients eat:

Breakfast

- Two whole eggs, two egg whites, spinach and peppers, and an apple
- Protein shake, a banana, and a serving of peanut butter (my favorite!)

- Serving of plain oats, strawberries, protein powder, and a serving of pecans
- Leftover sirloin steak, a serving of walnuts, and blueberries

Lunch

- Leftover meat from dinner, salad with one tablespoon of olive oil/balsamic dressing
- Can of lentil soup, apple, and one serving of almonds (one of my favorites)
- Turkey and ham sandwich on double-fiber bread (or just the meat), an orange, and carrots

Snack

- Protein shake, an apple, and maybe a serving of cashews
- A low-fat cheese stick or two and a banana

Dinner

- Chicken breast or lean chicken thigh, plain baked potato, and broccoli
- Sirloin steak, green beans, arugula salad with a serving of blue cheese and olive oil
- Salmon, sweet potato, and grilled zucchini

Be mindful of your portion sizes and eat slowly.

Even if you eat a healthy diet, it's still possible to eat too much. The easiest way to avoid this is to practice mindful and slow eating. Basically, you think a little more about your eating behavior before and during meals.

When serving food, ask yourself "Do I really need this much?" When eating, stop halfway through the meal and ask "How much more do I need to eat to be satisfied?"

Put your fork down between bites and chew thoroughly. Give yourself some time to enjoy your meal. This is something that I've struggled with personally, and after teaching it to others, it has helped me stay leaner and happier.

Another way to practice mindful eating is to avoid distractions at mealtime, like watching television or surfing the Internet. Sit down with your family and discuss the day. My wife and I traveled recently to Paris, and when we went out to dinner, we always finished our meals faster than everyone else. They were all talking and laughing in between bites. This is a great thing to practice.

Mindful eating is one of the tougher habits to learn, and my patients generally need a support group or a coach to help them fully master this. (You'll learn more about support groups and coaches in FLP Step #8.)

Janet's Story: Mindful Eating Made the Difference

Janet was a sixty-two-year-old woman who wanted to lose about fifteen pounds to help with her arthritis and knee pain. She loved walking, but she couldn't walk very long without excruciating aches. Her diet was healthy, so I suggested she try some of the mindful eating techniques above. She thought they were silly but gave them a shot.

In four months, she lost those fifteen pounds and is now able to walk three miles per day without knee pain.

Cook most of your own meals.

One of the single most important yet overlooked tricks for getting leaner is to cook more. If you can cook or learn to cook, your odds of being successful with this program just went up tenfold. The more meals you consume at home, the more likely you are to lose weight. Eating at restaurants makes it harder to lose weight for the following four reasons:

- Most restaurant foods have many "hidden" calories. A sandwich from Panera might include four hundred calories just from bread and still fail to fill you up. A large slice of pizza might have an extra five hundred calories depending on how much oil and cheese is added. You can't always tell how many calories prepared food has by looking at it.
- Most restaurant labels are wrong, often by a wide margin. Even if you carefully track your calories, you could be five hundred or one thousand calories off because the caloric estimations were inaccurate.
- Not all restaurants have healthy or lower-calorie options. If you never learn to prepare your own meals, you're stuck with whatever you can get.
- Most restaurant portions are two or three sizes larger than "normal" portions. You're likely to eat more because you're served more.

If you've never cooked before or aren't confident in your skills, start with something easy like scrambled eggs. If you really hate to cook, you can always use a meal delivery service, like Blue Apron or Plated, but this cost can add up quickly. Regardless, I suggest you try to eat at least 80 percent of your meals at home, preferably more. In other words, look at eating out as a treat, not your main source of food.

Speaking of treats...

Strategically indulge in treats.

Not only is it okay to have some dessert every now and then, it's a good thing. One of the reasons many people fail to lose weight is they overly restrict themselves. They think they have to give up chocolate or ice cream or doughnuts forever, and they end up breaking their diet one day and overeating. Then they quit.

When you get a craving, have a small portion of dessert or junk food or alcohol, and move on. It's much easier to keep your portions of junk food reasonable when you're eating an overall healthy diet and eating mindfully. Another good tip is to get the premium version of the dessert (e.g., high-quality dark chocolate instead of a run-of-the-mill candy bar). This way you will really enjoy it. I also tend to shy away from "healthy" desserts, like cakes and pies that replace flour with protein and use sugar substitutes. They never taste as good as the real thing.

The Next Step: Tracking Your Diet

If these strategies don't work for you, or if you want to guarantee that you'll lose weight, you may need to track your diet. Let me say that tracking is not a substitute for healthy eating behaviors. It's an additional tool to add more precision to your diet.

Generally, I don't recommend tracking calories unless the aforementioned methods aren't working, or you simply love monitoring your diet. When you count calories, you still must eat a high-quality diet, stay mindful of portion sizes, and indulge on occasion. But some folks can't lose weight by changing their habits and eating mindfully. If that's true for you, you may have to track your diet.

Second, the most important rule of weight loss is that you must be able to maintain the changes you're making. If you're making progress without tracking, I suggest you continue what you are doing for as long as you can. If your weight loss stalls or you start to regain weight, consider tracking your calories.

To track your diet, follow these steps:

Set a calorie target for the day. The easiest way to set your calorie target for weight loss is to multiply your body weight in pounds by ten to twelve. If you're a woman or a less active person, choose the lower range of ten to eleven; if you're a man or a more active person, choose the higher range of eleven to twelve.

Let's say you're a sedentary woman who weighs 170 pounds. Your math would look like this: 170 × 10 = 1,700 calories. You'd want to eat about 1,700 calories a day to lose weight.

If you're a 250-pound man with an active job, like a laborer, your math would look like this: 250 × 12 = 3,000 calories. You'd want to eat about three thousand calories per day to lose weight, give or take.

There are more complicated calculators out there, but all of these equations are just starting places. You'll have to adjust your diet as you go anyway to adjust for changes in body weight and how much energy you expend, so don't worry too much about the exact number. If you switch from a physically demanding job like construction work to an office job, you won't need as many calories. For example, if our man from the previous example switches to a less-demanding job, three thousand calories per day might be higher than our guy needs. He could probably cut back to twenty-five hundred calories, and he'd lose weight even faster.

Set your macronutrient (protein, carbohydrate, and fat) targets. After setting your total calorie intake for the day, you want to set a protein target. The easiest way to do this is to aim for about 0.75 to 1.0 grams of protein per pound of body weight per day. Our 170-pound woman would consume about 130–170 grams of protein per day; our 250-pound man would aim for about 190–250 grams of protein per day. The recommendations are based on the best available evidence, and they're the same for men and women. Aim to get close to this number every day. If you can't eat this much protein every day at first, that's fine. Just try to eat close to about thirty grams of protein per meal on average.

You can make this process even easier by using an app like MyMacros+ to set your macronutrient intake. You enter your desired percentage of carbs, fat, and protein, and the app tells you how many grams of each to eat per day. Some apps have barcode scanners, although hopefully most of the foods you choose will come from the produce section—and have no barcodes.

To use this type of app, adjust the macronutrient percentages to hit your protein target. For example, protein has four calories per gram, so if your protein target is two hundred grams per day, that's eight hundred calories from protein. If your total daily goal is two thousand four hundred calories and two hundred grams of protein, then 33 percent of your calories (eight hundred calories) will come from protein.

You can adjust your percentages of carbs and fat, which will depend on your personal preference and possibly your lab results. A typical breakdown will be around 30 percent protein, 40 percent carbs, and 30 percent fat. Here are my carb and fat recommendations:

- Make fat at least 10–15 percent of your calories. Any lower than that tends to cause much greater hunger and hormonal disturbances, especially for women.
- However, it's generally best to have fat comprise no more than 40 percent of your calories. Any more than that and you'll probably eat too many total calories (except for some situations, like when consuming a very low-carbohydrate diet).
- If you have a fasting glucose level of over one hundred milligrams per deciliter and/or a hemoglobin A1c of 5.7 percent or higher, opt for a lower carb intake of around 20 percent of your total calories. (This is a rough guideline; some of my patients with type 2 diabetes and prediabetes who exercise need a slightly higher percentage of carbs.)
- If you are active and have normal glucose levels, feel free to eat a higher percentage of carbs. This is especially true if you want to excel at my workout plan in the next chapter.

Track your calorie and macronutrient intake throughout the day. There is little point in setting specific calorie and macronutrient targets unless you track them consistently. The easiest way to do this is with a nutrition tracking app like MyFitnessPal, Lose it, MyMacros+, or FitDay. Enter the foods and amount you ate in your app, or write it down so you can enter it into your computer later.

To be precise, use a food scale and high-quality measuring spoons and cups. Measuring your food will help you be more accurate than if you eyeball your portions. I thought I knew what a serving of pasta was, but when I started measuring my foods, I realized I was eating twice as many servings as I thought!

Check your calorie and macronutrient numbers throughout the day. Are you short on anything? If you're low on protein, be sure to add more at your next meal. If you've eaten more calories than you intended, plan to cut back in later meals.

You may not hit your targets exactly, and you may be off the first week or two. With a few weeks of practice, though, you'll find it easy to achieve the percentages you want.

Frank's Story: Using Technology to Lose Weight

Frank, a forty-seven-year-old engineer at NASA, was worried about his triglycerides, which were creeping up. His waist was now forty-one inches, compared to the thirty-two inches it was in college. Frank told me he was eating a lot of protein and vegetables and trying to eat mindfully, but the weight wasn't budging. He even joined a gym with little result. I suggested he try MyMacros+ on his smartphone.

Being an engineer, Frank thought the numbers, calculations, and technology were really cool. He lost over twenty pounds within four months just by tracking his calories and macronutrients. His waistline is now smaller than forty inches, his triglycerides are back to normal, and he still uses the app today!

Five Tips to Combat Hunger and Stick to Your Diet

Many people think that if they aren't hungry, they aren't working hard enough to lose weight. It's true that you may get a little hungry sometimes while dieting, but that shouldn't be the norm. Here are five effective tips I use with clients to help them avoid or deal with hunger:

Tip One: Plan or prep your meals ahead of time.

This can be as simple as keeping a grocery list of what you plan to eat, or as specific as writing out exactly what and how much you're going to eat at each meal. Some people take this a step further and prepare their meals ahead of time for the day or week.

That's not necessary, but you should have a general idea of what you're going to eat later that day. Otherwise, it's too easy to eat whatever is tastiest or most convenient. Have a basic plan, and if you want to be more specific, such as deciding what you'll have for lunch before you head to the restaurant, go for it.

If you know when you'll get hungry during the day, be proactive and eat a small snack before that happens. For example, I have an apple and a protein shake around 3:00 p.m., a couple hours before I head home from work. It keeps me from attacking the fridge and pantry when I get home.

Tip Two: Keep fruit on hand as a quick snack.

You will generally eat whatever is most convenient. By keeping fruit or other healthy, low-calorie snacks on hand, you'll be much less tempted to go for M&M's or honey-roasted peanuts. Put a bowl on your counter or kitchen table, and fill it with oranges, apples, bananas, or whatever fruit you like. When you get low, fill it back up. You'll be surprised at how much easier it is to get in fruits and vegetables and pass up other snacks when they're in sight. (I learned this trick from Brian Wansink, author of *Slim by Design*. I highly recommend his book for more tips like this one.)

Tip Three: Eat slower.

Yes, I mentioned this earlier, but I am going to say it again. Eating more slowly helps your brain realize how much you've eaten so you can stop when you've consumed a reasonable number of calories. Thirty-seven-year-old Kathy lost over thirty pounds this way. I take some of my patients to lunch to chat about nutrition, exercise, and life—and to see how they eat. Kathy had admitted to having issues with her eating speed in the past, but when we got together for lunch after her weight loss, she had barely eaten a third of her food as I was finishing!

In between bites, we would converse, and she would put her fork down. It was amazing to see, especially since I was scarfing my food down like I had a trough in front of me. Her weight loss was not an accident. She learned a new habit and stuck with it.

Tip Four: Try protein and meal replacement shakes.

An easy way to keep your calories lower while increasing protein and keeping you full is to replace one of your meals with a protein shake. There are whole diets based on this method where you start off a rapid weight-loss plan with all of your meals as shakes. If a patient is having trouble with portion control or food quality at a particular meal, it's often helpful to replace that meal with a protein shake.

For example, have a protein shake for breakfast instead of a muffin and a high-calorie latte, and you'll cut calories and get in much-needed protein. You can do the same with lunch or dinner. Look for a protein shake or meal replacement drink that has at least twenty to thirty grams of protein, and consider adding nuts, fruit, and even vegetables (if you have a good blender) to it. These add calories, but also make you feel full longer.

My favorite protein powders are those made from whey, casein, milk, and egg, but you can also choose vegan options like rice, pea, and soy protein.

Tip Five: Consider medicine.

It's possible that you may still struggle with hunger even if you use these fives tips. If that's the case, consider using certain medications to help you adhere to your diet. (We'll cover these in more depth in chapter seven.)

Very Low-Carb and Very Low-Fat Diets: What You Should Know

Diets that severely limit carbs or fat do work, but not in the way most people think. They each eliminate a macronutrient—carbs in one case, fat in the other—which automatically lowers your calorie intake. Interestingly, studies show that both of these diets are equally effective. Guess what determines your success on each? You got it—*adherence*.

If you choose one of these diets, you must follow it closely and consistently. That's the only way it will work long term. If you want to follow one of these diets, it's important to work with a coach or physician to pick the diet that's right for you.

Very Low-Carbohydrate Ketogenic Diets

Many of my patients have blood sugar issues, and lower-carb diets tend to work better for them.

Most benefits of a low-carb diet come from eating fewer calories and losing weight. When they lose weight, their insulin sensitivity improves, which improves their blood sugar. Either way, a very low-carb diet that includes fewer than fifty grams of carbs per day may also help with appetite regulation.

A "ketogenic diet" is one where carbs are restricted enough that your body begins to produce fuel from another source—ketones. Basically, a "ketogenic diet" is just a fancy term for a *very* low-carb diet, usually fewer than about 30–50 grams per day. I don't promote this diet to most patients because it's so hard to stick with. It may be worth a shot, however, if you're having trouble controlling your appetite with the FLP plan and don't want to take medicine.

A very low-carbohydrate, high-fat ketogenic diet may help promote satiety, which can help you stick with it long term. However, if you opt for a very low-carb diet, you'll eat less protein than I recommend. Instead of the macronutrient breakdown I gave earlier, your diet will consist of about 20 percent protein, 5 percent carbs, and a whopping 75 percent fat. Get most of your fat from olive oil, avocado oil, and nuts instead of butter and cream to reduce saturated fat.

A word of caution: I have had many patients do this diet with great results, but some develop very high levels of LDL, or "bad" cholesterol, and apolipoprotein particles, which are another marker of cardiovascular health. This is likely due to the high amount of saturated fat they're consuming. That's why I promote healthier sources of fat like olive oil and nuts. Some people say high levels of LDL are harmless, but there's no evidence to support this. If you eat a very low-carb, high-fat diet, monitor your cholesterol with a physician familiar with this kind of diet.

Very Low-Fat Diets

Low-fat diets were pushed as the best way to eat starting in the 1960s and '70s. They can be healthy and effective for weight loss, but most people don't follow them correctly. Instead of focusing on the whole, nutritious foods I recommend, they eat highly refined and/or sugary foods, which happen to be low in fat. These foods are easy to overeat, and people often consume far more calories than they realize. This is why many people who go on low-fat diets don't lose weight and may even gain weight.

If you choose a low-fat diet, you will want to get most of your calories from nutritious, low-fat whole-food sources. This means a diet that includes many plants, a few lean protein sources, and very few refined foods. Your percentage of calories from fat ends up being less than 30 percent, and some propose that the percentage be kept much lower than that.

Dr. Garth Davis, a well-known bariatric surgeon, is a strong proponent of low-fat vegan diets. Dr. Davis wants his patients to change their diets so they don't even need surgery. He pushes high amounts of plants, which fill people up without all the calories. This high-fiber diet also works well for people with blood sugar issues.

So what's the takeaway? Either of these diets can work for you—if you stick with it. That's the most important factor to consider before choosing one.

Rick's Story: A Very Low-Carb Diet Worked for Me

Rick, thirty-one, dove right in with a very low-carb, ketogenic diet after I mentioned it to him, and he lost thirty pounds in four months. He didn't struggle with hunger, and his energy increased so much that he is now able to exercise daily, something that many believe isn't possible with a low-carb diet. Rick's blood sugar and blood pressure went from on the border of needing medicine to perfectly normal.

Very low-carb diets don't work for everyone, but for some people, like Rick, they're a perfectly good option.

Should You Take Supplements?

Many of my patients ask about weight-loss supplements and want to know whether they should take them. If a supplement claims to "burn fat" or help with fat loss, in a word, the answer is "no." Some current "hot" supplements include raspberry ketones, garcinia, and green coffee beans, but there are no safe supplements that will make your body burn fat.

Supplements can be a convenient way to hit your calorie and macronutrient goals. If you're running short on time, for example, a protein shake can help you hit your protein goals for the day.

Protein and meal replacement shakes can be extremely helpful for meeting your protein goals, even when you're busy. Many studies show that meal replacements often improve weight loss, especially when they're substituted for higher-calorie meals. The added protein can help you build muscle and recover from workouts. Protein powders, especially made from whey, may also help improve blood pressure and blood-glucose control.

I suggest you limit protein powders and meal replacements to one or two a day. Rely on whole foods for most of your meals and snacks. There are some other supplements that can be helpful for maintaining your health. If you're interested in learning more, go to my website, www.FatLossPrescription.com.

Keeping Perspective: Think Progress, Not Perfection

I've found that many people think they need to find the ideal combination of foods or macronutrient ratios or supplements before they can lose weight. The truth is that the people who lose the most weight and keep it off focus on making consistent progress. They find ways to eat fewer calories than they burn, day after day, and lose weight. Continuously work on your eating choices, and you'll be able to do the same.

How you eat is only one third of the FLP program. How you move is the next part, which we'll talk about in the following chapter.

3

The Fat-Loss Prescription Guide to Activity

T HE PREVIOUS CHAPTER introduced you to the first three FLP steps on how to eat. In this chapter, we'll talk about the three steps that refer to how you move:

FLP Step #4: Exercise regularly.
FLP Step #5: Lift weights *and* do aerobic exercise.
FLP Step #6: Make movement a part of your daily routine.

If I had one thing to prescribe to all of my patients, it would be exercise. Heck, you already know exercise is important. At one point you may have even enjoyed it. But now it seems like every time you try to start a new workout program, you get bored and quit.

Why? There are several problems with most weight-loss exercise programs:

- They fail to take into account your personal preferences.
- They focus only on burning calories and making you sweat, but they ignore other benefits.
- They force you to do too much too soon.
- They feel like punishment.
- They promise massive weight loss, which isn't likely.

The FLP program takes a different approach. There are only two rules to exercising. You must (1) pick something you enjoy and (2) do it consistently. Everything else is a bonus.

Studies have shown that a combination of strength training and "cardio," or aerobic exercise, is your best bet for weight loss and health. Each type of exercise provides unique benefits you can't get from the other. Strength training increases your muscle mass and strength and makes your bones and connective tissues stronger. Aerobic exercise does a better job of improving your cardiovascular function and blood pressure. It also tends to burn slightly more calories (which still matters) than strength training.

So how does exercise help with weight loss? If your only goal is fat loss, exercise doesn't make a huge difference. Most studies indicate that the relatively small amount of exercise most people are willing to do doesn't have a dramatic impact on weight loss. It helps you lose slightly more fat than if you don't work out, but most of your progress will be thanks to changing your diet.

But exercise is extremely important for two main reasons:

- Studies have repeatedly shown that exercise makes it much easier to *maintain* your new weight. One reason people gain weight back so quickly after dieting is they don't make exercise a habit.
- Exercise, especially strength training, helps you maintain muscle, which comes with a huge number of long- and short-term health benefits.

There are other benefits too, like improved mood, lower chance of cardiovascular disease, better sleep, and more self-confidence—plus you'll fit better in your clothes.

But you have to do something that you can make a habit. So start by choosing an activity you enjoy. Think of the kinds of exercise you like to do or that you enjoyed when you were younger. Walking? Playing tennis? Throwing a Frisbee with your dog? Swimming? Cycling? Splitting wood, lumberjack style?

It doesn't matter what kind of exercise you choose as long as it keeps your heart rate slightly elevated for a continuous period of time. This doesn't mean you should be gasping for breath after a few minutes. It means exactly what it sounds like—you're working just a little harder than you would normally, but not so much that you want to collapse at the end.

Aim to Exercise Every Day

Your goal is to get in a short workout—say thirty minutes of light to moderate exercise—every day. Moderate exercise is the equivalent of a brisk walk. For the best results, aim for a more structured workout several times per week as well. Walking after every meal is an easy way to get in exercise time, and you don't have to do all thrity minutes at once if you don't want to.

Should You Run?

Considering running to help you lose weight? Keep this phrase in mind: "You should lose weight to run, instead of running to lose weight." If you're carrying a lot of excess weight, running can be hard on your joints. If you're committed to running, make sure to get properly fitting shoes at a running store, where staff can recommend the best brands for you. Start off slowly, briskly walking before transitioning to jogging. The "Couch to 5k" program (www.c25k.com) is free and lets you gradually ramp up to running.

Include Weight Lifting as Part of Your Program

Most workout programs focus only on how many calories you burn. Burning calories is nice, but you also need to maintain (and build, if possible) muscle mass. Don't worry, ladies—you will not get big muscles from lifting weights, I promise.

Running, Zumba, and swimming are all great forms of exercise, but they do little to maintain muscle mass as you lose weight. When you lose weight, your body will try to break down fat, muscle, and connective tissue to burn as energy. The less muscle you lose, the more fat your body must burn instead.

Maintaining muscle also means you burn more calories all day, as muscle burns slightly more calories than fat. Lifting weights and stressing your muscles beyond how you normally do also sends your body the signal that you still need your muscles, making it less likely to break down muscles for energy.

Lifting weights can burn a significant number of calories and does improve cardiovascular health, but that's not the main goal here. The real goal is to maintain muscle mass and make you stronger.

Here are the two exercise plans I provide patients:

Dr. Spencer's "Planet Fitness" Fat-Loss Workout Plan

Okay, so you don't *have* to do this at Planet Fitness, but a lot of my patients go there because it is so cheap, and it has the basic equipment you need. With this plan, you'll use workout machines and won't need to hire a trainer to get started. (I highly recommend you get a trainer in the near future, but that's often not practical at first.)

This is a starter plan, similar to the exercise recommendations of the *American College of Sports Medicine*, that is meant to get you in the habit of exercising, while giving you some great initial results. That said, some of my patients stick with this plan for months or years and continue to get great results.

If you're already doing something more advanced than this, first off, kudos! Second, move on to the next plan.

With this plan you will lift weights three days per week, doing two to three sets per exercise and eight to twelve repetitions.

You'll perform these main exercises each workout:

- Machine bench press
- Machine overhead press
- Machine back row
- Machine overhead pull-down
- Leg press

If you have time, you can perform these accessory exercises:

- Leg curl
- Leg extension
- Bicep curl
- Triceps extension

In addition to three days of strength training, you'll do aerobic exercise three to four days per week (or more if you wish).

Don't be scared. You only need to do the equivalent of thirty minutes of brisk walking or cycling. "Brisk" means you should be able to talk—but not sing—while exercising. You should be breathing a little faster than normal without huffing and puffing.

That's it! Follow this plan if you're a beginner or new to exercising.

Dr. Spencer's Advanced Fat-Loss Workout Plan

If you're working out already or want a more challenging exercise regime, try my Advanced Fat-Loss Workout Plan. If you exercise more often or more intensely, you'll get better results in terms of weight loss, muscle building, and improvements in health markers like blood pressure. With this plan, you'll be training much more and see even more benefits.

For results and to avoid injury, it's important to perform these exercises correctly. If you're not sure how to do them, check out the videos on my website that demonstrate them (www.fatlossprescription.com/exercises).

The Advanced Fat-Loss Workout Plan includes two components: lift weights four days per week and do four to six cardio workouts each week. Here's what your weight-lifting routine will look like. Shoot for two to three sets per exercise and eight to twelve repetitions per set:

Day 1: Upper body
- Dumbbell bench press
- Dumbbell back row
- Dumbbell military press
- Dumbbell pull-over
- Dumbbell skull-crusher (triceps extension)
- Dumbbell alternating curl
- Hanging knee raises

Day 2: Lower body and bike
- Barbell squat or split squat or leg press
- Conventional or sumo deadlift
- Stiff-legged deadlift
- Leg curl
- Thirty to sixty minutes of moderate-intensity biking. You can swap this for twenty minutes of higher-intensity work, like interval training, where you up your intensity to an uncomfortable pace for a minute and then recover at an easier pace for a minute, and repeat.

Day 3: Aerobic exercise only
- Thirty to forty minutes light intensity exercise (e.g., jogging or using the elliptical trainer)

Day 4: Upper body
- Barbell bench press (can switch to incline or decline)
- Barbell row or machine row
- Barbell military press
- Lat pull-down or regular pull-up (can be assisted)
- Back extension
- Side raise
- Optional cardio: twenty to thirty minutes on the rowing machine

Day 5: Cardio only
- Long, easy-paced sixty-minute bike ride

Day 6: Lower body
- Dumbbell Bulgarian split squat (if this is too difficult, a regular split squat is fine)
- Dumbbell deadlift
- Dumbbell stiff-legged deadlift
- Dumbbell farmer's walk
- Leg curl
- Plank

Day 7: Cardio only
- Moderate-intensity workout (e.g., jogging or using the elliptical trainer) for forty minutes

Cardio Guidelines

You want to get *at least* thirty minutes of cardio each time it's scheduled in your plan. If you can get sixty minutes, that's even better. You want your pace to be fast enough that you can still talk, but only with effort, and in one- or two-sentence bursts. This is tougher than the brisk walking pace in the first workout plan.

If you're a patient of mine, ask me to accompany you to the gym so we can work on these exercises. If you can afford a personal trainer (which I highly recommend), that's even better.

FLP Step #3: Make movement a part of your daily routine.

Before the 1900s, most people didn't do much formal exercise. Instead, they stayed extremely *active*. They chopped wood. They carried groceries home from the store. They walked across town instead of driving. All of these little movements added up throughout the day.

You've heard that you need to "move more and eat less." Well, "move more" doesn't just mean exercise. All of the moving we do during the day counts. In fact, the movement you do outside of formal exercise can be just as important, if not more so, than your structured workouts.

When people want to lose weight, they often start by eating less. They also start working out several hours per week. So far, so good. But they don't realize that their total amount of daily movement may have decreased. They may be sitting more or doing less, even rationalizing that they exercised already so they don't have to move as much. In some cases, this lack of activity is enough to negate the calorie deficit they've created, and it can halt weight loss.

All the little movements you do in the course of a day fall under the blanket term of "nonexercise activity thermogenesis," or NEAT. Basically, NEAT is a fancy way of saying "small movements that aren't considered formal exercise." Petting your cat. Holding a coffee cup. Tying your shoes. Opening your car door. Those are all small movements, yet they still burn calories. While none burn that many calories by themselves, the total can be surprisingly high.

In one study, researchers found that fidgeting (like jiggling your legs) while sitting burned about 50 percent more calories than just sitting. Standing while fidgeting burned almost 100 percent more calories than sitting. Walking at an easy pace burned nearly 200 percent more calories than sitting.

We're talking fairly small numbers. If you burn five calories a minute sitting, 100 percent more is only ten calories a minute. However, even minor increases in your energy output throughout the day can make a big difference.

Think of it this way. There are 168 hours in a week. If you follow the exercise program in this book, you'll do weights and cardio for about five hours a week. If you sleep eight hours a night, that's another 42 hours. So 61 hours of your week are tied up in sleeping and training.

That leaves 107 hours in the week for you to move more, even a little bit. Compare that to just five hours a week of formal exercise, and you can see how much opportunity there is for burning more calories.

Here are five ways to get more activity into each day:

Use a device to track your activity. Tracking your daily movement can be extremely motivating and eye-opening. Tools like Fitbits, Bodybugs, Jawbones, and most pedometers monitor how many steps you take and how many calories you burn throughout the day.

These devices don't accurately measure the calories burned through formal exercise like cycling and running. But they do measure how much you're moving *outside* of regular exercise.

While these tools aren't 100 percent accurate, you can still use them as motivation. For example, if your device says you normally walk four thousand steps a day, you can try to walk four thousand five hundred or five thousand steps a day. Seeing the numbers can give you the push you need to stay more active.

Use a standing desk. A standing desk lets you work while standing, but you don't have to have an actual standing desk. Try putting your computer on a box on your desk or on a cabinet so that you can work standing for periods of time. Standing for much of your workday can burn as many calories as a sixty-minute bike ride or run.

Ease into standing more; try standing for thirty minutes or an hour at a time, and increase gradually.

Get up from your desk more often. Even if you don't use a standing desk, set a timer to ring every forty-five minutes. When it goes off, get up and walk for five minutes. The latest research shows sitting all day may have some very negative health consequences. Get up every forty-five minutes to combat this problem, and you'll probably feel more energetic and focused at work.

Take the stairs whenever possible. A flight of stairs is basically a bunch of body weight step-ups, so use escalators and elevators as little as possible.

Park farther from your work building. Parking even one hundred yards from your workplace can make a big difference in your calorie burn. And you'll probably save time because you're no longer trying to get the "best" parking space.

Another reason to make daily movement a habit is that it's more flexible than formal training. If you're traveling for work, for example, you may not be able to get to the gym as often, but you can still sneak in a lot of activity.

Mary's Story: Taking More Steps

Mary, thirty-eight, has polycystic ovarian syndrome, or PCOS, which makes it harder to lose weight. She had lost twenty pounds but then hit a plateau. I convinced her to get a Fitbit to see how many steps she was taking per day.

Mary was only taking about two thousand steps, so I gave her the goal of hitting five thousand steps per day. Within a few weeks, she was consistently hitting her goal. We then went up to seven thousand five hundred and finally ten thousand steps. She was able to break through her plateau and lose another eight pounds, which gave her the motivation she needed to add more exercise and continue losing weight.

4

How You Live: The FLP Steps
to a Healthier Lifestyle

S O FAR WE'VE talked about how to eat and how to move. Now let's talk about how you live. The last three FLP steps are:

FLP Step #7: Get more, and better quality, sleep.
FLP Step #8: Get support from others.
FLP Step #9: Find ways to handle emotions that don't involve food.

Let's look at sleep first. When it comes to weight loss, diet and exercise get all the attention. In many cases, however, sleep can be just as important. When you don't get enough sleep, you generally make poorer eating decisions and are less likely to exercise or move a lot during the day.

Studies have shown that sleep-deprived people tend to eat more calories during the day than those who get enough sleep; they also tend to lose more muscle mass while dieting.

Sleep deprivation affects your overall health, too. People who don't get enough sleep generally have shorter life spans than better sleepers. They also have a higher risk of type 2 diabetes, metabolic syndrome, and high blood pressure.

Finally, when you're short on sleep, you just don't feel good. You're more likely to be depressed, irritable, moody, and you're less likely to make good decisions.

Most people don't get the seven or eight hours of sleep a night that studies show you need for optimal health. Even shorting yourself by an hour or two a night can have a negative impact on your insulin sensitivity and quality of life. One night of poor sleep won't ruin your health, but chronic sleep deprivation can cause major problems.

FLP Step #7: Get More, and Better, Sleep

There are no "hacks" or shortcuts when it comes to sleep. You need to get enough, period. But there are research-proven strategies for falling asleep faster and improving your sleep quality.

Go to bed and wake up at the same time every night. This trains your body to fall asleep and rise automatically and makes it easier to get a good night's rest. An erratic sleep schedule generally makes it harder to fall asleep, and leaves you feeling groggy in the morning. Aim to go to bed and get up at roughly the same time every day.

Wake up without an alarm if possible. If you get enough sleep the night before, you generally shouldn't need an alarm in the morning. Your body will rest as long as it needs. If you need an alarm clock, I recommend a sunrise clock, which uses light instead of noise to awaken you. This may help your natural circadian rhythm. For most of human evolution, we used light to wake up, not an alarm. Humans also sleep in cycles, and there's some evidence that waking up in the middle of a cycle may cause more grogginess. If you use an alarm, your chances of waking up in the middle of a sleep cycle are higher. If you use light, it's possible that you'll have a better chance of waking up between cycles.

Sleep in a completely dark, cool, and quiet room. Exposure to light causes the release of stimulating hormones that keep you awake. That's great in the morning when you're trying to get up, but the opposite of what you want when you're going to bed.

Put dark curtains over your windows and turn off all electronics in the room. Minimize noises or choose a white-noise machine or fan, which drowns out sounds that can keep you from sleeping.

A cool room will enhance your sleep, too. A few studies have shown that 66 to 68 degrees Fahrenheit is generally more conducive to sleep than normal house temperatures, which are around 70 to 72 degrees.

Shut off computers and televisions at least an hour before bed. Light tells your brain to stay awake. Looking at the television, phone, tablet, or computer before bed will make it harder to fall asleep. You may want to try the software f.lux, which darkens your computer screen automatically at night.

Limit caffeine intake to before noon (preferably before 10:00 a.m.). Caffeine can stay in your system for quite a while and may disrupt your sleep when consumed later in the day. Stick to consuming it before noon to prevent it from interfering with your sleep. (I generally don't drink caffeine after 10:00 a.m.) Drinking alcohol at night can also mess with your sleep cycles. If you regularly drink more than two alcoholic beverages before bedtime, think about cutting back.

Shift Worker? What You Can Do about It

Night shifts or rotating shifts that go from days to nights frequently can make it very hard to get into a healthy sleep cycle. If you have a job like this, your best bet is to try to find another one. If that's not possible, you'll need to add more structure to your diet and get the best sleep you can.

If you have to do shift work, try these tips:

- Darken your room as much as possible.
- Plan or prepare your meals ahead of time so you'll have them ready when you get hungry.
- Pack some healthy snacks to combat hunger during your shift, which is more likely with shift work.
- Exercise regularly. This will make it much easier to fall asleep.
- Create a flexible, yet structured diet that will work around your schedule.

Identifying Common Causes of Insomnia

Having trouble sleeping? I know I have in the past. If you're dealing with insomnia, you should talk with your doctor to try to figure out the cause. *Short-term insomnia* is when you have trouble sleeping at least three times per week for fewer than three months. This is often due to life stressors and hopefully resolves after the stressor is gone. *Chronic insomnia* is when you have trouble sleeping at least three times per week for more than three months.

Although it's tempting to wait for insomnia to get better on its own, it's best to see your doctor in the beginning before it gets worse. When I treat patients with short-term insomnia, I make sure they're following the steps I recommended earlier in this chapter. Sometimes I recommend one to three milligrams of melatonin thirty to sixty minutes before bed. Melatonin is a hormone related to sleep patterns and can *sometimes* help combat insomnia.

If that doesn't work, we'll discuss medicines like zolpidem (Ambien) and cognitive-behavioral therapy to treat insomnia. I don't recommend over-the-counter sleep aids very often, as they can make you groggy the next day.

Jen's Story: Working around a Shift Work Schedule

Jen is a thirty-four-year-old nurse working rotating shifts who was trying to lose weight. We both knew the shift work was a factor, but she couldn't just quit her job. We worked on various nutritional habits, including counting her calories and macronutrients, but her weight loss stalled.

Jen told me she had no issues with her first meal (usually a protein shake) or the meal she brought to work, which was typically a salad with meat. However, she admitted that when she came home exhausted and hungry, she'd rummage through her pantry and fridge to satisfy her cravings.

Jen had already mastered some basic healthy-eating steps like having more protein and eating slower, but she kept her late-night cravings to herself because she was embarrassed. Once she told me about her late-night eating habits, we created a plan.

She started eating an orange at work before she left for home. That took the edge off her hunger so she didn't feel the need to ransack her pantry. She had very little time to cook before bed, so we found a decent grocery store nearby that had healthy prepared foods and a salad bar. She built her last meal from options at the grocery store, and if it was closed when she got home, she'd have a simple meal of lentil soup with Greek yogurt and berries.

With just a few simple changes, Jen was able to completely eliminate those late-night binges. Jen lost twenty-five pounds and has kept the weight off for over three years now.

Sleep Apnea: What to Do If You Have It

Many people walk around with almost unbearable levels of fatigue and no idea what's causing it or what to do about it. I screen all of my patients for Obstructive Sleep Apnea (OSA) because it can have such a horrible effect on people's lives, and it's far more common than most realize. Only about 8 percent of the US population has sleep apnea, but among obese and overweight people that number rises to about 75 percent.

Sleep apnea prevents your brain from getting enough oxygen when you sleep. Then you feel terrible during the day, and your blood pressure, blood sugar, and risk of heart disease all increase.

If you have the following symptoms, make sure you talk to your doctor about the possibility of having OSA:

- You gasp or stop breathing in the middle of the night. (Ask your spouse or partner if this happens.)
- You snore.
- Your neck is over seventeen inches (forty-three centimeters) in circumference and you're a man, or over sixteen inches (forty centimeters) and you're a woman.
- You never get restful sleep, and you're extremely tired in the morning.
- You fall asleep easily during the day, such as in your chair at home or even at a stoplight.

Your doctor may recommend that you undergo a sleep study, where you spend the night in a hospital or lab and doctors monitor your sleep quality. Depending on your results, they may recommend a continuous positive airway pressure (CPAP) machine, which is a mask similar to what fighter pilots wear that pushes air into your lungs.

The idea of a CPAP machine doesn't sound fun, but all of my patients who have used it felt like a million bucks after they started wearing it. They get better sleep, which makes it easier to stick to the FLP steps and lose weight. As you lose weight, you may be able to stop using the CPAP machine, but it's a very helpful tool in the meantime.

Mark's Story: Better Sleep = More Weight Loss

Mark, a forty-year-old schoolteacher, came to me for help losing weight. He had pre-diabetes and high blood pressure, which he was taking a diuretic for. Mark knew he had to lose weight, but he lacked energy. We worked on a few nutrition and exercise habits, but his weight didn't budge. He admitted he was only doing them about half of the time.

We checked Mark's thyroid and testosterone, and both were normal, though his testosterone was a little low. I suggested he do a sleep study because I was nearly certain he had obstructive sleep apnea. He admitted to snoring and sometimes gasping for air while sleeping; plus, his neck was nineteen inches around, and he was visibly tired all of the time. He could barely write his lesson plans without falling asleep at home.

Mark didn't want to do the sleep study because he didn't want to spend the night attached to a bunch of wires with people watching him. On top, he said that even if he had sleep apnea, he wouldn't wear the CPAP machine.

I bargained with him, and promised that even if he need the CPAP machine, I could eventually get him off it. This was a gamble on my part because not everyone who loses weight can stop using a CPAP machine, but I needed a Hail Mary at the time.

Mark had severe sleep apnea, and the doctor prescribed a CPAP machine. Within a month, he came in looking like a new man. He said his energy had improved fivefold, and with that energy, he was able to work on nutrition and exercise. His weight started coming down quickly. He lost fifty pounds within six months, and his CPAP was adjusted to a lower level. His testosterone has increased again, and he's still working to eliminate the need for the CPAP entirely, but he is thankful that he decided to get it.

FLP Step #8: Get Support from Others

This step may surprise you, but I suggest you join a community of people who also want to lose weight. Community is one of the most underrated yet important aspects of behavior change, especially with weight loss.

Weight is often a touchy subject. You may not be comfortable talking about it, and it's easy to fall into the trap of thinking that you can do it on your own. But studies have shown that when people want to make a permanent change in their lives, they need a close group of supportive friends to make it really stick.

Starting a habit is great, but even if you pick something sustainable, like doing twenty minutes of exercise per day, things will come up that interfere. Maybe a relative will die. Maybe you'll go on a trip and slip out of your routine when you come back. In many cases like this, people abandon their new habits and fall back into old behaviors.

Friends can form a set of guardrails around your behavior. When you start to go off the road, they set you back on track. This doesn't mean your friends should yell at you when you eat cookies or drag you to the gym. That's not helpful. Supportive friends don't even need to give you advice to have a positive impact. Just being around people who are working toward similar changes is often enough to make it easier for you, too. When you see other people creating healthier habits, you start to believe that it's possible for you. There's a reason Alcoholics Anonymous works so well for so many people—it creates a tight group of supportive people all working to help each other change.

However, if many of your friends and family are practicing the behaviors you want to avoid, spending time around them might make it harder to change. What to do? Join an online group of people who are working toward similar goals. Studies have shown that people generally get better results with behavior change when they have someone checking on them online.

To make a permanent change—the kind that's resistant to stress, traveling, and boredom—you must believe that change is possible. Spending more time around people who are working toward the same goals as you helps you believe that. That's why I created an online support group for patients and FLP followers. It's a place to surround yourself with others going through the same journey.

About half of my patients join the group, and the other half decide to do the program alone. The half that joins typically loses twice as much weight as the half that doesn't. Dr. Sherry Pagoto, a researcher at the University of Massachusetts Medical School, has found similar results in some her studies looking at private social-media groups. Those in the groups help each other lose weight more than their friends or family do. It is quite amazing.

Take Action—Right Now

I have a request. If you haven't done so yet, I want you to join my free online support group. It will only take a second. Just go to www.FatLossPrescription.com, enter your email address, and I'll send you a link to the private support group on Facebook. We let people join in batches, so it may take a week or so for your request to be accepted. When you see we're accepting new members, mention that you're reading this book, and you'll get moved to the front of the line.

Should You Consider a Coach?

Finally, when we're talking about the importance of support, I know that self-help books (this one included) can only go so far. Along with the online group, you may want to consider hiring a weight-loss coach who can be there for you even when your doctor, friends, family, and support group are not.

Some studies show that coaches do not have to be highly trained psychologists to be effective. Good coaches have many traits in common, but your coach's main goal should be to help you ingrain the FLP steps. Your coach should also have empathy and compassion for your struggles and shouldn't berate or yell at you (unless you want that).

If you're interested in hiring a health and weight-loss coach, visit www.DrSpencer.com/coaching.

FLP Step #9: Find ways to handle emotions that don't involve food.

Studies have shown that how we handle our emotions is directly related to our likelihood of maintaining a healthy weight.

Many people, especially those who are overweight, use food as a coping mechanism for other life stressors. If their boss is being a jerk, if they're going through a breakup, if they're dealing with financial problems—food becomes a very tempting distraction and escape.

That's what emotional eating is—using food as a way to cheer yourself up or distract yourself from another stressor. We've all probably done this to some degree, but for many people, it can become a crippling habit. In one study, 70 percent of people who regained a significant amount of weight after a diet reported that they often ate for emotional reasons instead of true hunger.

One of the best strategies for dealing with emotional eating is to work with a skilled therapist. There's no shame in seeking help. However, most people want to work on this problem by themselves first. Here are some strategies for dealing with emotions in ways that don't involve food:

Acknowledge that emotional eating is an issue for you. Many people who suffer from emotional eating don't realize that's what they're doing, and that may be why they haven't been able to do anything about it. Or they've been eating emotionally for so long that it feels normal.

Only you can decide if you're eating due to actual physical need or because you're trying to deal with other emotional issues. So think about it. Start that discussion with yourself.

Create an environment that makes it easier to make good decisions, even when you're bored or stressed. Everyone deals with stressful, draining experiences throughout the day. Some days aren't so bad, and other days you want to stab someone with a pencil. You may be able to control your emotions during the day, but when you come home, the temptation to splurge on a box of cookies will likely still be there. Instead of trying to will yourself through these situations with discipline, a better solution is to create an environment that requires less willpower to make good decisions:

Keep smaller portions of junk food (or none) around the house.

Keep junk food in places that are harder to get to, such as putting ice cream at the bottom of your freezer.

Leave fresh fruits and vegetables in plain sight, or better yet, prepared and ready to eat in the fridge.

Have another activity planned for when you get home so you aren't stuck in the kitchen, brooding about the day or thinking about what to do next.

Have other hobbies and projects that you can work on. Food is one of the most convenient sources of entertainment. All you have to do is buy a bag of snacks and you're good to go. Better yet, you can sit in front of the TV or computer and eat while watching a movie or playing a game.

But, as you know, that's also a great way to gain a bunch of weight and waste a large chunk of your day. Instead of using food to fill your time, have other hobbies and interests that you can work on when you're not at your job. Think of what you used to do when you were a kid. Are there any other projects you've been promising yourself you'll start, but you feel like you never have time? Maybe you have been interested in learning a new instrument? Taking a martial arts class? Reading more? Building cabinets? Or painting a room of your house?

Use constructive projects that challenge and entertain you to fill your time instead of food. The best hobbies are the ones that make you lose track of time while you're doing them.

Keep a journal of how you're feeling. Awareness is one of the most effective habits for dealing with emotional eating. Before you can change the way you respond to stress or boredom, you have to become aware of the triggers. A simple way to do this is to write down every time that you feel stressed or bored and a few ideas *why* you feel that way. Don't be judgmental or hard on yourself, just write down what you're feeling so you can look at the situation more objectively.

You can't necessarily control your emotions at all times, but you can improve how you respond to those emotions. Use the above steps to cultivate awareness for how you feel, identify the triggers that cause you to eat emotionally, and reprogram how you respond in the future. It'll take time, but the benefits will pay off.

5

Tracking Your Progress and
Maintaining Your New Body

Y OU'RE FOLLOWING THE FLP steps, but there's one more important task ahead of you—tracking your progress. You wouldn't run a business without keeping track of your profit and costs. You wouldn't plan a road trip without making sure you had enough gas to get to your destination. Numbers matter; keeping track of the ones that matter most for weight loss can be extremely helpful.

Research proves that people who track their weight-loss progress get better results. Don't worry about the time involved or what to track; it doesn't have to be time-consuming. Track a few metrics, or statistics, and you'll know how you're progressing and be more motivated to stick to the program. Keep the following tips in mind when monitoring your results:

Weigh yourself regularly. Multiple studies prove that people who weigh themselves regularly get better results than those who don't. You'll be more aware of your weight and likely to be more careful about your diet-and-exercise plan.

But don't get too fixated on the scale. Your scale weight isn't the only thing that matters, and small fluctuations aren't a big deal. You want to have a general idea of how much you weigh, so focus on trends, not small shifts. Weighing yourself two to three times a week seems to work best for most people.

Track your results in a spreadsheet, a journal, or a nutrition-tracking app, or simply write your weight on a piece of paper next to the scale. You might also consider a cool Wi-Fi scale, such as the ones made by Fitbit or Withings, which will record your weight automatically and send the data to your phone or computer. If you obsess over the scale (like many of my patients), tape a piece of paper over the display and check your weight weekly; you'll see trends, not daily spikes.

If the number on the scale isn't moving, it may be for the following reason(s):

- If you're a woman, it may be due to hormonal changes during your menstrual cycle, which affect water retention.
- Maybe you ate more the day before and haven't digested the food yet.
- Maybe you ate more salt the day before and are retaining extra water.
- Maybe you ate more carbs than usual over the last few days and are retaining extra water.
- Maybe you didn't drink as much water—or you drank more water.
- Maybe you drank more alcohol than normal, which can cause large amounts of water loss.
- Maybe you weighed yourself at different times of day.
- Maybe you wore different, heavier clothes that added a pound or two.
- Maybe you gained muscle and lost fat at the same time.

Get the idea? There are many reasons why the scale may not budge despite the fact that you're doing everything right. This is why daily or even weekly fluctuations aren't important. It's the overall trend that matters.

Nearly all of my patients have times when the number on the scale doesn't move—yet their clothes fit better, and they look different. People *love* numbers, but it's important to remember that they are not the only indicator of progress.

Bridget's Story: You Can't Always Trust Your Scale

Bridget, one of my online followers, is a thirty-four-year-old bank manager. She weighed around 255 pounds when I first talked to her. Bridget was following my program to a T. In two months, she was excited to have lost eleven pounds. A week later, she stepped back on the scale to see that her eleven pounds were back. She freaked out, understandably.

Her clothes felt looser, and her friends and family had noticed a major difference, especially in her face and waist, yet her scale said she was back to her original weight. I convinced Bridget that the scale is not the only measure of progress; photos, the way your clothing fits, and circumference measurements are also great tools. I told her maybe something was wrong with her scale, or she had a fluctuation in water weight. Within a week, the eleven pounds fell back off, and she continued getting lighter from there. Crisis averted. She has now lost a total of twenty-five pounds.

Aim for a Reasonable Rate of Weight Loss. Your goal is to lose weight steadily, not necessarily quickly, and keep it off forever. Faster isn't always better. More consistent is better. Start conservatively, and change the plan if you plateau. If you're struggling with hunger, consider talking to your doctor about medications that may help. (See chapter seven for more on weight-loss drugs.)

For most people, a loss of one pound per week is a good goal. That's usually doable with the diet and exercise plan in this book, and it's easy to remember. You may lose significantly more or slightly less than that amount—some people lose as little as half a pound per week, others lose as much as four pounds per week. Much of that will be water weight, but much of it will be fat, too. If you're losing less than half a pound per week, you may want to change your diet-and-exercise plan to cause faster weight loss.

Take progress pictures. Progress photos keep you honest. It's easy to forget how much progress you've made, but losing thirty pounds over several months will show up in pictures. You'll likely be amazed at how big of a difference it appears to be. I suggest you take progress photos, even if you don't share them with anyone else.

A few tips for good photos include the following:

- Use the same camera every time. Phone cameras tend to be easiest.
- Use the same lighting each time.
- Take the pictures at about the same time of day. First thing in the morning often works best.

Take circumference measurements. You want most of the weight you lose to be fat, not muscle. If you only measure your weight, you won't know the difference. But if you're losing weight and your circumference measurements are going down, it's likely you're losing fat. It's also possible that your weight may not change for a while, although your circumference measurements keep going down. That means you're probably still losing fat while maintaining (or gaining) muscle.

Wrap a tape measure around the following areas:

- Waist. Locate the top of your hip bone on either side with your hand. Wrap a tape measure around your waist at those two points.
- Thigh. Measure the distance between the top of your hip bone and the top of your kneecap with a tape measure. Mark your skin with a pen halfway between those two points. At the spot where you marked your skin, wrap the tape measure around your thigh.
- Upper arm. Locate the bony tip of your shoulder and run a tape measure from that spot to the bony tip of your elbow (with your arm relaxed at your side). Mark your skin halfway between those two points. Measure the circumference of your arm at the spot you marked. You may need someone to help with this measurement.

(You only need to take thigh and arm measurements on one side of your body, but it should be the same side for both measurements).

Record those numbers on a spreadsheet, an app, or a piece of paper, and use them to track your progress.

Keep a journal. Finally, keeping a journal of your thoughts and feelings while you change can be extremely eye-opening. When you get frustrated, when you want to quit, when you regret starting the diet, when you want to beat yourself up, write it down. One of the goals of losing weight is to improve your confidence and happiness. When your journal entries look more positive over time, that's a good sign.

Should You Consider More Advanced Body-Fat Testing?

If you want to get really precise, you can opt for more advanced body-fat testing. Dual X-ray absorptiometry (DXA) is the most accurate. You lie on a table while a machine sends low-powered X-rays through your body, which determine how much body fat and lean body mass you have. DXA machines are usually used for bone mineral density instead of body-fat testing, so confirm that the doctor's office performs body-fat testing before making an appointment.

The BodPod is another popular method that uses air displacement to measure body-fat changes. Hydrostatic weighing is similar to the BodPod, except it uses water instead of air.

These methods are fancier, and more expensive, but they aren't necessarily more helpful than regular weighing and circumference measurements. The DXA, BodPod, and hydrostatic weighing all have fairly wide error margins, meaning they could still read well above or below your actual body composition.

Some doctors' offices offer BIA (bioelectrical impedance analysis) too. BIA devices can be highly inaccurate but may show fat-loss trends during your journey. You can buy a BIA device for home use, but they can give wildly inaccurate readings. Bottom line? You're better off, in my opinion, sticking with regular weighing and circumference measurements.

Maintaining Your New Body

After you've reached your goal weight, what happens? You keep up the same routine and continue to follow the FLP program for life. If there's one thing you take away from this book, it's that the only way you'll be able to maintain your new body is by changing your habits. You've learned about the nine FLP steps and how to put them into action. Now, how do you keep those healthy habits going for good?

One of the biggest mistakes people make is jumping into a new program, making too many changes at once, and then getting discouraged after they can't stick to the plan. That's why most diet plans only work for a few months before people quit. Low-carb diets, high-carb diets, low-fat diets, and virtually every other kind of diet tend to work for about the same length of time. They all get about the same results because people cannot adhere to them long term.

Yet most people struggle far more with maintaining their new weight than they do with losing weight. In other words, people can often lose a significant amount of weight, but they tend to gain it back quickly. That's why about 93 to 98 percent of dieters ultimately fail.

You want to make sure that you can maintain your new behaviors. If you cannot see yourself performing a particular habit for the long term, then break it into a smaller change. For example, if you don't think you could eat protein at every meal for the next few months, then start by eating protein at two meals a day. If you don't think you can work out thirty minutes every day, start with twenty, or even ten, minutes a day.

Before you start any diet, exercise program, or habit of any kind, ask yourself, "Am I 90 percent confident I can maintain this behavior for the next month?" If the answer is "yes," then go for it. If the answer is "no," then consider scaling that habit back. Consistency is key.

Fuse Your New Habits to Old Ones

One of the easiest ways to build a new habit is to combine it with something you already do.

Say you want to consume more protein. If you add it to every meal, it makes it easy to remember because you're already eating several times a day.

This is why I recommend people walk after their meals. If you take even a short walk after every meal, it's much easier to remember to do it. If you're trying to exercise more, I suggest doing it first thing in the morning. You have to wake up every day anyway.

Change Your Environment

You learned in chapter one that your environment has a huge impact on your behaviors. If you always have candy lying around or your freezer is filled with processed foods, you'll eat that most of the time. A television in your bedroom makes it more likely you'll start watching a movie when you should go to sleep. And if you want to swim for exercise, but the only pool is a thirty-minute drive across town, you're less likely to go.

Small changes to your environment can have a big impact on your actions. For example, if you leave a fruit bowl out, you're likely to eat more fruit. If you leave running shoes by the door, you're more likely to go running. If you keep a book by your bed, you're more likely to read instead of watch television.

If you want to learn more about how to make these changes, I highly recommend Brian Wansink's book *Slim by Design*. It details how making small changes to your surroundings will make it easier to stick to good habits.

Katie's Story: A Coach Made the Difference

Katie, a forty-six-year-old patient of mine, came to me for weight-loss advice. She was about 210 pounds at five feet six inches but wasn't taking any medications and had no medical issues. She lost twenty pounds in two months without a problem, but all of a sudden, Katie's weight started creeping back up. Even though she continued to see me monthly, she gained back about ten pounds. She enjoyed the Facebook support group but wanted more.

I suggested Katie join the VIP section of the support group, where she could work with a coach to provide more consistent accountability and guidance. Within a few months, she lost the weight she had regained as well as another fifteen pounds. Katie is still working with her coach to achieve her weight-loss goals.

Weight loss isn't a destination or deadline. It's a process. The FLP steps are not only essential for weight loss, they're essential for weight *maintenance*.

Don't get sucked into the trap of trying to lose weight as fast as possible. There's a reason most of the contestants on shows like *The Biggest Loser* gain back much of the weight they lose. They rushed the process, and they couldn't stick to their new lifestyle.

Start with small, effective changes, and build from there. You'll lose weight. It might not be easy all of the time, but with patience, you will achieve your goal.

Part 2

When the FLP Steps Aren't Working

USE THE FLP program with all my patients. That doesn't mean they all get the exact same plan, and that's part of why this works so well—they each get a customized program they can adhere to.

Sometimes, however, people need a little extra help. As effective as these steps are, not everyone makes as much progress as others. This doesn't mean the system doesn't work; it's just further proof that everyone faces different challenges. The next part of this book shows you why some people have a harder time losing weight than others and what to do about it.

6

Conditions and Medications That
Can Interfere with Weight Loss

OR MANY PEOPLE, following the FLP steps is all it takes to lose weight. Others, however, may struggle with weight loss even while adhering to the steps. People in the latter group may have a medical condition or disorder that increases risk of weight gain, or they may have developed a disorder that can result from weight gain (or both).

Six Medical Conditions That Can Affect Weight Loss

I get a lot of questions from health coaches and personal trainers who have clients who can't seem to lose weight despite eating "one thousand calories a day" or otherwise sticking to a rigid diet plan. They could have a thyroid issue. They could have had a rare kind of brain surgery that changed the way their bodies respond to hunger and deposit fat.

But most of the time, the people are eating more and moving less than they think they are. If you know you're following the FLP steps and still can't lose weight, you may want to talk to your doctor about the following conditions:

Hypothyroidism (low thyroid)

Hypothyroidism is the main medical condition people think of when they aren't losing weight. Your thyroid plays a huge part in determining your metabolic rate, so thyroid issues *can* have an impact on your weight. But while many people *think* their inability to lose weight is due to their thyroid, often that is not the case. Low thyroid affects up to about 10 percent of the general population.

And it doesn't necessarily cause dramatic weight gain. (In medical school, I found out that I have a form of hypothyroidism, Hashimoto's thyroiditis, or autoimmune thyroiditis. Even though I was hypothyroid, I was still very lean, healthy, and athletic.)

Symptoms of Hypothyroidism:

- Fatigue
- Unexplained weight gain
- Constipation
- Dry skin
- Foggy memory
- High cholesterol
- Feeling cold
- Low heart rate

If you have most of these symptoms, check with your doctor about getting tested for hypothyroidism.

Cushing's Syndrome (a.k.a., high cortisol or hypercortisolism)

This condition is relatively rare but can cause unexplained weight gain. It is most commonly due to prescribed corticosteroid medicines like prednisone for various conditions (a.k.a., iatrogenic Cushing's syndrome). So if you're taking corticosteroids, be aware that you might experience weight gain and the symptoms below. However, some folks may have tumors that cause the body to produce too much cortisol, which is extremely rare (only a few cases per million people per year).

Symptoms of Cushing's Syndrome:

- Increased fat around the face (a round-face appearance called "moon face"), abdomen, and neck (called "buffalo hump")
- Striae, which look like dark purple stretch marks usually located on the belly but also possible in other places
- Easily bruised, thinning skin
- Darkened area around neck and armpits, called acanthosis nigricans
- Facial hair on women (hirsutism)

If it is possible you have Cushing's syndrome, your doctor can test for it or refer you to an endocrinologist.

Hypogonadism (a.k.a., low testosterone or "low T," men only)

If you're a man with low testosterone, you may find it harder to lose weight. Your doctor will want to figure out the cause by asking you questions, running tests, and retesting to avoid lab errors or misinterpretation.

Symptoms of Low Testosterone:

- Low libido (sex drive)
- Decreased ability to get and/or keep erections
- Decrease in facial hair (less shaving)
- Feeling weak and tired/decreased energy levels
- Depression

One of the most common causes for lower testosterone in men today is obesity itself (along with insulin resistance, metabolic syndrome, and type 2 diabetes). If this is the case, losing weight will actually help bump up your testosterone. You may decide to opt for testosterone replacement therapy even if the cause is obesity, because it will help you build muscle, lose weight, and feel better.

This is one of those "chicken-and-egg" situations. In a perfect world, no one would need testosterone replacement therapy, and everyone could up his testosterone through lifestyle changes alone. On the other hand, testosterone therapy may make the process much easier. You'll have to talk about this with your doctor.

Polycystic Ovarian Syndrome (PCOS, women only)

The relationship between PCOS and weight gain and obesity isn't perfectly straightforward. Only around half of women with PCOS are overweight. But if you are overweight, it's worth talking about with your doctor.

Symptoms of PCOS:

- Irregular periods, no periods, or infrequent periods
- Facial hair (hirsutism)
- Weight gain
- Acne
- Blood sugar or insulin issues (high fasting blood sugar and insulin/insulin resistance)
- Cholesterol issues (high total and LDL cholesterol, low HDL cholesterol, and high triglycerides)

There is an overlap between these symptoms and those of Cushing's syndrome, but PCOS is much more common than Cushing's syndrome. Your doctor will want to test for other possible causes of these symptoms, like hyperandrogenism (high testosterone in women), which is why it is important to discuss your symptoms with your physician.

Binge-Eating Disorder

While many physicians and health coaches don't recognize this as a disorder in their clients, it is a real issue that needs to be addressed. Around 50 percent of those with binge-eating disorder are obese, and this can become a major barrier to weight loss if left unaddressed.

To meet the criteria for binge-eating disorder, you must experience at least three of the following, with episodes at least once a week for three months:

- Eating more rapidly than normal
- Eating until feeling uncomfortably full
- Eating large amounts of food when not feeling physically hungry
- Eating alone because of embarrassment by the amount of food consumed
- Feeling disgusted with oneself, depressed, or guilty after overeating

If you're struggling with binge-eating disorder, talk with your doctor. I generally recommend cognitive behavioral therapy with someone specially trained in dealing with patients who have binge-eating disorder. Selective serotonin reuptake inhibitors (SSRIs) along with anticonvulsants like topiramate and zonisamide have been used with some success for binge eating. Lisdexamfetamine (Vyvanse), a stimulant used for attention deficit hyperactivity disorder (ADHD) is also approved for this.

Can Menopause Cause Weight Gain?

Patients often ask me this question. Weight gain can occur around menopause, but for now the only solution to combat this is a solid lifestyle plan similar to the FLP steps. It's unclear Looking at the research, it's unclear whether hormone replacement therapy (HRT) helps with weight loss. However, HRT may help reduce the visceral fat stored in your abdomen. Either way, a good lifestyle plan is probably the most effective choice.

So Why Can't I Lose Weight?

There are other rare genetic syndromes and issues that cause weight gain, so if you feel like there is something else going on, find an obesity specialist who can determine the culprit, which may include the following:

Genetics. There are a number of genetic syndromes such as Prader Willi and single gene defects like MC4R deficiency that can hinder weight loss. Generally these conditions are found at a young age and must be addressed by an obesity, endocrine, or genetic specialist. Currently, the best way to work around your genetics is with the steps in this book, and with medicine and surgery if necessary. Those are things you should speak with a doctor about.

Hypothalamic obesity. While rare, a tumor, surgery, or trauma in the brain can result in this kind of weight gain. In chapter one, I discussed the faulty wiring in the brain that can cause excess hunger and excess fat storage. This is an *extreme* version of that.

Judy's Story: HRT Wasn't the Answer

Judy, at fifty-four, had gone through menopause a couple of years prior. She had gained about ten pounds so far on her 5'4" body and wasn't happy about it. She'd heard that HRT would help with weight loss, but she had no menopause symptoms like hot flashes or vaginal dryness. Her sex life was great. I explained that HRT was to address those symptoms, not weight loss.

We went over her nutrition-and-exercise plan, and it was apparent that Judy was still eating the same way she did in her twenties. She was lucky she hadn't gained more weight. I explained that she could make some simple lifestyle changes to bring her weight down and prevent future weight gain, and I asked her to start a resistance-training program to keep her bones strong. Judy started eating more protein and vegetables, cut out some junk food, and started going to the gym. She lost those ten pounds and gained strength at the same time.

Medications That Affect Your Weight

In addition to the medical conditions listed in this chapter, many common medications can affect your weight. Most of them cause weight gain while others can cause weight loss. I've listed them briefly here. In chapter seven, you'll find more information about how these drugs influence weight loss.

Warning: Don't stop any of these medicines without speaking to your physician first.

Depression Medicines:

- Paroxetine (Paxil)
- Amitriptyline (Elavil)
- Nortriptyline (Pamelor)
- Mirtazapine (Remeron)

Mood Stabilizers and Anticonvulsants:

- Valproic acid (Depakote)
- Gabapentin (Neurontin)
- Pregabalin (Lyrica)
- Carbamazepine (Tegretol)
- Vigabatrin (Sabril)
- Lithium

Antipsychotics

- Olanzapine (Zyprexa)
- Clozapine (Clozaril)
- Quetiapine (Seroquel)
- Risperidone (Risperdal)
- Ziprasidone (Geodon)
- Aripiprazole (Abilify)

Diabetes Medicine

- Glyburide (DiaBeta)
- Glipizide (Glucotrol)
- Glimepiride (Amaryl)

- Nateglinide (Starlix)
- All insulins
- Pioglitazone (Actos)
- Rosiglitazone (Avandia)

Blood Pressure Medicine

- Metoprolol (Toprol-XL)
- Atenolol (Tenormin)
- Propranolol (Inderal)

Birth Control

- Medroxyprogesterone acetate (Depo-Provera)

Steroids

- Prednisone
- Dexamethasone
- Hydrocortisone
- Inhaled steroids

Antihistamines

- Diphenhydramine (Benadryl)
- Hydroxyzine (Vistaril)
- Loratadine (Claritin)
- Fexofenadine (Allegra)
- Cetirizine (Zyrtec)

Jan's Story: Changing Medicines May Help

Jan is a fifty-seven-year-old woman with type 2 diabetes. She came to see me about her diabetes because her usual doctor was booked. Reviewing her chart, I saw that she had gained about thirty pounds since starting the medicine glipizide ten years prior, and her blood sugar was still uncontrolled, with a hemoglobin A1c of 8.5. She said she felt tired. I asked her if she'd be interested in changing her medicine and working on a few nutrition changes and exercise habits to improve her energy, blood sugar, and weight. She thought about it for a second and said, "Sure!"

Jan had no exercise or nutrition plan in place. We discussed taking a walk after each meal, filling her plate with green vegetables first, and replacing her glipizide with metformin. She said metformin had made her stomach upset in the past, but she agreed to try the extended-release formula only at night. She stuck to her lifestyle changes and tolerated the new medicine well. We did this for a few weeks to make sure the new medicine would work in the long term. It did, and she stuck to her new lifestyle changes as well.

I then asked whether she would consider taking liraglutide (Victoza), an injectable medicine that would help her lose weight and lower her hunger levels. She was very hesitant because she didn't want to inject herself daily, so we agreed on dulaglutide (Trulicity), which is similar but taken only once a week.

After a few more months of these medicines (and starting a strength-training program to help with blood sugar control and bone strength), her sugar levels were already out of the diabetic range (A1c of 6.1), and she had lost the thirty pounds! She continues to work out and improve her eating to hopefully someday get off the injection completely.

7

What You Should Know about
Medicine and Surgery for Weight Loss

T HE FLP STEPS are enough for most people to lose weight. However, some of my
patients need extra help, whether through medication, surgery, or both. This
chapter will give you an overview of the options currently available.

Yes, every medicine and surgery has risks, but so does staying overweight. Keep in
mind that medications and surgeries will be more effective when combined with the
FLP steps.

Medications Can Help with Weight Loss

If you struggle with hunger, there are medicines that can help control cravings and
further suppress appetite. I use them with patients who have a tough time adhering
to the FLP steps. They're all approved for those with a BMI over 27 and comorbidity,
or another medical condition, such as high blood pressure, diabetes, or sleep apnea.
They're also approved for adults with a BMI over 30. (None are approved for use during
pregnancy, and weight-loss medication should be stopped immediately if you find out
you are pregnant.)

These drugs work on different areas of the brain and affect people in different
ways. You may have to try several different medications before you find the one that

works best for you. Note that none of these "burn" fat. They work by reducing appetite or lowering the absorption of calories. Some are meant to be used long term, and others should only be used for shorter periods. You'll want to talk with your doctor about whether a drug is appropriate for you before trying one.

Long-Term Weight-Loss Medications

Phentermine/Topiramate Extended Release (Qsymia)

Qsymia, approved in the United States in 2012, combines two drugs that have been out for a while—phentermine and topiramate. Phentermine has been used for medical weight loss for decades and works as an appetite suppressant. Topiramate has been used for seizures and migraines for quite some time, but helps reduce appetite as well, affecting a different area of the brain. This drug combination causes a more robust drop in appetite with fewer side effects than higher doses of either drug alone.

Qsymia is one of my go-to weight-loss medicines because you only have to take it once a day, and it has a powerful effect on weight loss. People who take it also seem to improve their blood pressure, blood sugar, and other weight-related issues. There's also a trial underway to see if this drug reduces people's overall risk of death.

Qsymia comes in two maintenance doses and two titration doses, which means the dose can be increased as needed over time.

Topiramate causes birth defects. If you are a fertile woman, you should use contraception while using it, and your doctor may recommend a pregnancy test every month.

Lorcaserin (Belviq)

This is another long-term weight-loss medicine approved in the United States in 2012. It works on a special serotonin receptor in the brain and reduces your hunger differently than other drugs. Lorcaserin may also help lower blood sugar more than most other weight-loss drugs.

Belviq is taken twice a day and may cause less weight loss than Qsymia. This is a serotonin-like medicine, so be careful taking other serotonin-modulating medicines like antidepressants. Some doctors allow patients to take both, but be careful to avoid a condition called "serotonin syndrome," which can be very dangerous.

Naltrexone/Bupropion Extended Release (Contrave)

This combo medicine was approved in the United States in 2014 as a long-term obesity medicine. The mix of bupropion and naltrexone work together to reduce hunger and cravings. Both medicines are approved for substance-abuse issues like tobacco and alcohol, and they work in the addiction part of the brain. I tend to use this medicine with patients who crave certain foods.

One big drawback to this medicine is that you have to titrate, or increase the dose, up from one pill per morning all the way to two pills in the morning and two pills at night. This can be a lot of pills! The medicine causes about the same amount of weight loss as the other medicines on this list. Don't take this medicine if you take opioids or narcotics for anything, because the naltrexone will prevent them from working.

Liraglutide (Saxenda)

This is the newest long-term obesity medicine approved in the United States, and it's actually a higher dose of medicine that was already approved for diabetes (Victoza). Sazenda is an injection that works through a different hunger-related pathway in the brain. I've used this medicine with my patients in the form of Victoza (the one approved for diabetes) with very good results, but I have not used the higher doses for weight management yet. Using this higher dose may help appetite regulation even more, but it also may cause side effects such as nausea.

Orlistat (Xenical)

Orlistat was originally approved in the United States in 1999 for long-term weight loss and is available over the counter. It blocks fat absorption, which means you digest fewer calories when you eat. Although the data shows the medicine works very well, I don't use it with patients often. The side effects from the malabsorption of fat are steatorrhea (fatty or greasy stools) and even fecal discharge when passing gas (commonly referred to as "shart"). It's easy to see why I don't prescribe this often.

Short-Term Weight-Loss Medicines

Phentermine

Phentermine has been approved since 1959 for treating obesity, but only for twelve-week increments or shorter. It works as an appetite suppressant and is cheap and effective, which is why many doctors prescribe it for twelve weeks or longer. If I want to prescribe phentermine, I try to stick with Qsymia, which is approved for long-term weight loss, but if the patient cannot afford it, I will prescribe phentermine alone for longer than twelve weeks.

Some physicians pair this with a separate prescription of topiramate to mimic the combo medicine Qsymia. I have prescribed Qsymia many times with good success, but one of its most common side effects is insomnia.

Diethylpropion

This is another weight-loss medicine approved for short-term (twelve weeks) use that decreases appetite. It likely won't be as effective as phentermine, but some physicians still prescribe it. This drug doesn't last as long in the body as phentermine, so some physicians prescribe this in patients who struggle with insomnia. While I haven't prescribed it, other obesity-medicine physicians have had good success with it.

Phendimetrazine

This is another medicine approved for only twelve weeks and works similarly to those above. I have not prescribed it so far.

Crystal's Story: A Medication Made It Easier to Eat Fewer Calories

Crystal is a thirty-three-year-old patient who said she was doing everything right but wasn't losing weight. She was eating mostly whole foods. She was counting her calories and claiming to eat only 1,200 calories a day. She was running, lifting weights, and sleeping well. So what was wrong? She didn't have a medical issue and wasn't binge eating or snacking constantly.

I thought she might be underreporting her food intake. Many people eat twice as much as they think they are, so it's possible she was eating 2,400 calories or more.

I thought Crystal might benefit from trying a weight-loss medicine, so I went with Qsymia because she'd had a hysterectomy and was not at risk for getting pregnant.

After a month, she lost six pounds, more than she had lost in the past four months. The medicine helped her eat less, and she said it was much easier to eat 1,200–1,500 calories per day. After a year, she had lost another fifty pounds. It's been two and a half years so far, and she's kept the weight off.

Weight-Loss Surgery: Another Option

Sometimes, the best lifestyle modifications, medicines, and support teams aren't enough. Bariatric surgery is an option to consider if you have a BMI over 40 or a BMI over 35 along with a weight-related issue like high blood pressure or type 2 diabetes. Talk to your doctor about a referral to a good bariatric surgeon, if appropriate, if you've failed to lose weight with lifestyle changes and medicines.

Here is a brief rundown on the types of bariatric surgery available:

Adjustable band

A surgeon puts a band around the upper portion of your stomach, which reduces the amount of food it can hold and (hopefully) helps fight hunger. I honestly don't recommend this procedure. While it seems safer than other options and is reversible, its effects on weight loss are mild at best. I suggest you consider the other options listed in this chapter.

Gastric bypass

There are a few ways of doing this procedure, but the most common is called the "Roux-en-Y," which is named for the surgeon who invented the procedure and the shape of the surgery. The surgeon basically makes a little pouch out of your current stomach and then realigns your intestines. This prevents you from absorbing all the calories you consume and reduces your appetite.

This procedure does have drawbacks. You will want an awesome surgeon because this type of surgery has a higher risk of death and other problems than the other bariatric surgeries. It is irreversible, and the malabsorption resulting from the procedure may mean you need vitamin and mineral supplements.

THE FAT LOSS PRESCRIPTION:

Gastric sleeve

This newer procedure involves cutting out a large portion of your stomach, leaving it looking like a banana instead of a football. Like the band and bypass, the sleeve restricts food; it also affects your hunger hormones like the bypass. This option seems to be safer than the bypass, but we don't have a lot of data about how effective it is. Like the bypass, it's irreversible, and you may need to take extra vitamins and minerals afterward.

Other types of surgery

Recently two other procedures were introduced in the United States. One is called the VBLOC, in which a small transmitter is placed in your body near your vagus nerve. The transmitter is supposed to block appetite signals from your stomach to your brain; however, the weight loss seems minor, and none of my patients have tried this yet.

Another type of surgery was just approved while writing this book. During this procedure, called endoscopic balloon insertion, a balloon is placed through your mouth into your stomach. It fills up your stomach, which is supposed to make you feel fuller. There are two brands of balloons, ReShape and Orbera, and they are approved to be used for up to six months at a time. I have not referred any of my patients for this either.

If you're considering weight-loss medication or surgery, consider the risks and benefits before making a decision. Talk to your doctor, and don't be afraid to get a second opinion.

8

Taking Medication? A Closer Look
at Medicines and Weight Gain

A s YOU SAW in chapter seven, many common medications can affect weight loss by affecting appetite, fat storage, and energy levels. If you use any of the following medications, talk with your doctor about how they may affect your weight-loss efforts. And never change or discontinue any medication without talking to your doctor first.

Psychiatric Medications for Depression

Some depression medicines have side effects that can impact your body weight, including the following:

Tricyclic antidepressants

These drugs are used for depression, headaches, and other neurological pain issues. The biggest culprit in this class is amitriptyline, but nortriptyline is also associated with weight gain. Imipramine and desipramine are associated with less weight gain.

SSRIs (selective serotonin reuptake inhibitors)

These are commonly prescribed for depression and can cause weight gain. The biggest culprit here is paroxetine (Paxil), while citalopram (Celexa) and escitalopram (Lexapro) seem to be weight neutral. Fluoxetine (Prozac) and sertraline (Zoloft) may be associated with some weight loss in the beginning and are neutral in the long term.

SNRIs (serotonin-norepinephrine reuptake inhibitors)

This is a relatively new class of antidepressants. In general, these are weight neutral or may cause a small amount of weight gain, at most. These include venlafaxine (Effexor), duloxetine (Cymbalta), desvenlafaxine (Pristiq), milnacipran (Savella), which is only approved to treat fibromyalgia in the United States, and levomilnacipran (Fetzima).

Other drugs

Mirtazapine (Remeron) is sometimes used for depression and also for its specific side effect of weight gain. If you're taking it, talk to your doctor about potential replacements.

Bupropion (Wellbutrin) is generally my go-to antidepressant since it is the only one that shows consistent weight-loss properties. It isn't always effective for depression, however, and can cause side effects, but it is also part of a combination medicine called Contrave that's approved for weight loss.

To treat depression, I try to get all of my patients to see a psychologist who is trained in cognitive-behavioral therapy. People with mild depression may not need medicine; for others, I may recommend bupropion or at least pick the weight-neutral options as much as possible.

Mood Stabilizers and Anticonvulsants

I generally refer patients with bipolar disorder or epilepsy to a good psychiatrist or neurologist, and then I discuss their specialists' recommendations with them. Valproic acid (Depakote), gabapentin (Neurontin), pregabalin (Lyrica), carbamazepine (Tegretol), vigabatrin (Sabril), and lithium are all associated with weight gain, some more than others. However, these drugs may be necessary for your condition, so do *not* just stop taking them.

Lamotrigine (Lamictal), levetiracetam (Keppra), and phenytoin (Dilantin) are weight neutral. Topiramate (Topamax), zonisamide (Zonegran), and felbamate (Felbatol) are all associated with weight loss. (Like bupropion, topiramate is used in a combination medicine approved for weight loss. Zonisamide may also be approved in the future in a combination medicine for weight loss.) You may not be able to switch medications, but it's worth asking.

Antipsychotics

These drugs are among the worst offenders when it comes to weight gain, which is why they should not be used haphazardly. I rarely prescribe these unless I am in a pinch and cannot get my patient to a good psychiatrist. Not only do they cause weight gain, they cause insulin resistance, aggravate symptoms of type 2 diabetes, and worsen levels of LDL cholesterol.

Olanzapine (Zyprexa) tends to be the worst, followed closely by clozapine (Clozaril), quetiapine (Seroquel), risperidone (Risperdal), ziprasidone (Geodon), and aripiprazole (Abilify). Ziprasidone and aripiprazole cause the least amount of weight gain. These medicines are not necessarily interchangeable, and they should all be managed by a psychiatrist.

Diabetes Medicines

A few of these medications can cause weight gain, and switching to another can result in large amounts of weight loss. You may also be able to get off most of these medicines if you follow the FLP steps. Weight loss often eliminates obesity, which is linked to insulin resistance and type 2 diabetes.

Metformin (Glucophage/Glumetza)

Metformin is a diabetes medicine that is considered the best first-line medicine against type 2 diabetes. The drug appears to work by making your body more sensitive to insulin while telling the liver to suppress glucose production. It is cheap, safe, and associated with small amounts of weight loss.

Everyone who has type 2 diabetes should be on this medicine if possible, but some people can't tolerate the side effects such as diarrhea. You can try switching to the extended-release version to be taken at night or taking it with food. Glumetza is a special formulation of metformin that may decrease side effects as well.

GLP-1 agonists (Glucagon-like peptide-1)

Along with metformin, these are my favorite to prescribe for patients with diabetes because of their potent weight-loss and blood sugar lowering properties. These are injectable medications, but the needles are small, and the benefits are huge.

GLP-1 is a hormone produced in your stomach. It helps your pancreas make more insulin and less glucagon, which helps lower your blood sugar. GLP-1 also suppresses hunger signals in the brain and your rate of gastric emptying, the speed at which food leaves your stomach, to make you feel more satiated. When you have type 2 diabetes, your body doesn't make as much GLP-1 anymore; these injections help replace it.

The GLP-1 agonist I prescribe most is liraglutide (Victoza). This GLP-1 is associated with the most weight loss out of all of them, but it must be injected daily as opposed to weekly. If you don't want to inject yourself daily, I generally recommend dulaglutide (Trulicity), as it is associated with a good amount of weight loss and blood sugar lowering and comes in an easy-to-use weekly pen. Exenatide (Bydureon) is also fine but not as easy to use due to the preparation of the injection pen. Albiglutide (Tanzeum) is the least potent option. I don't use it with patients.

SGLT2 inhibitors (sodium-glucose cotransporter-2)

These are the newest class in type 2 diabetes medicines. They basically work by making you pee out more sugar, which means you are losing calories through your urine and not storing it as fat. This may sound weird, but the process lowers blood sugar and causes some weight loss. The medicines in this class include canagliflozin (Invokana), dapagliflozin (Farxiga), and empagliflozin (Jardiance). I have used all three with good success.

DPP-4 inhibitors (dipeptidyl peptidase-4)

These are another new class of diabetes medicines that are mostly weight neutral. They work by inhibiting an enzyme called DPP-4, which breaks down GLP-1. As you just read, GLP-1 helps your pancreas make more insulin and less glucagon, a hormone that increases the amount of sugar in your blood. GLP-1 also slows down gastric emptying and makes you feel fuller. Taking a DPP-4 inhibitor means you'll have more of your own GLP-1. The medicines in this category are sitagliptin (Januvia), linagliptin (Tradjenta), saxagliptin (Onglyza), and alogliptin (Nesina). I only use these medicines with patients who don't want to use GLP-1 agonists.

Sulfonylureas/Meglitinides/Secretagogues

I'm not sure why these medicines are prescribed anymore other than the fact that they're cheap. These medicines make your pancreas produce more insulin to lower your blood sugar, but they can cause weight gain. These drugs also have a higher risk of abnormally low blood sugar (a.k.a., hypoglycemia) than similar drugs. The worst offenders are glyburide (DiaBeta), glipizide (Glucotrol), glimepiride (Amaryl), and nateglinide (Starlix). There are other medicines that can actually help you *lose* weight and manage your diabetes.

Insulin

Insulin may be necessary if you are a type 1 diabetic, a type 2 diabetic who doesn't produce enough insulin anymore, or severely insulin resistant. Basal, or long-acting, insulin comes in lower doses and may have a lower weight gain associated with it. The long-acting insulins include glargine (Lantus/Toujeo) and detemir (Levemir). The short-acting, or bolus, insulins are lispro (Humalog), aspart (NovoLog), and glulisine (Apidra).

There is an intermediate-acting insulin called NPH as well as mixes of intermediate- and short-acting insulins (usually in a 70/30 ratio). The insulin that seems to cause the least amount of weight gain is detemir (Levemir), but my goal is to have my patients on the least amount of insulin possible, regardless of type. Using the FLP steps and alternative medicines, you may be able to lessen or even eliminate the need for insulin.

TZDs (thiazolidinediones)

These medicines actually cause fat gain, but I use them occasionally. They help to improve your insulin sensitivity, lower blood sugar, and make you more likely to store "good" fat (around your hips and thighs) and lose "bad" fat (around your middle). The two medicines in this class are pioglitazone (Actos) and rosiglitazone (Avandia).

Others

Other diabetes medicines include acarbose (Precose) and miglitol (Glyset), which prevent the breakdown of complex carbohydrates so you don't absorb as much sugar during digestion. They are weight neutral or may be associated with weight loss, but you have to take them at the beginning of each meal. Their biggest side effect is flatulence.

Bromocriptine (Cycloset) is a dopamine agonist that is approved for type 2 diabetes. It seems to work on increasing insulin sensitivity, but it's weight neutral. I haven't used it with any patients.

Colesevelam (Welchol) is a bile acid sequestrant (meaning it interferes with the absorption of fat), which was originally used for lowering cholesterol. It lowers blood sugar as well and is weight neutral. I have used it with a few patients.

Pramlintide (Symlin) is an injectable drug for both type 1 and type 2 diabetes that mimics the substance amylin. Like GLP-1, it is associated with lowered blood sugar and weight loss. It's expensive and must be injected before each meal. I have not prescribed this medicine.

Greg's Story: Losing Forty Pounds in Three Months

Greg is your classic blue-collar worker. Now fifty-five years old, Greg had gained seventy pounds, mostly around his belly, over the last twenty years. He only came in for a checkup every few years. At one appointment, his fasting blood sugar was 280 mg/dL, and his A1c was 11. For reference, both of those numbers are more than twice the recommended level for a healthy person.

I called Greg and explained that he needed to come back to discuss the results of his blood work. With a hemoglobin A1c level of 11 (over 6.5 is considered diabetic), some physicians would start with insulin right away. But he wasn't having symptoms of glucotoxicity, such as excess urination and tingling and numbness in the hands and feet, so I suggested he be very aggressive with lifestyle and noninsulin therapies.

Greg started on the FLP steps, and I put him on metformin XR/dapagliflozin (combo medicine called Xigduo XR) and dulaglutide (Trulicity). The results were nothing short of amazing.

In three months, Greg lost forty pounds and normalized his blood sugars (98 mg/dL with an A1c of 5.7). His clothes were basically falling off of him at his next appointment, and he had much more energy. Greg is continuing to follow the FLP steps and hopes to get off the dulaglutide and/or dapagliflozin as he loses more weight.

Blood Pressure Medicines

Obesity and poor lifestyle choices are often the causes of high blood pressure, and losing weight may eliminate the need for blood pressure medicine. There are multiple blood pressure medicines to choose from, and only a few are associated with weight gain.

Beta-blockers

Beta-blockers work by blocking the effects of adrenalin on your heart and blood vessels. This decreases your blood pressure but can also cause weight gain. Beta-blockers are still used after a heart attack and for heart failure and atrial fibrillation.

Commonly prescribed medicines in this class include metoprolol (Toprol XL), atenolol (Tenormin), propranolol (Inderal), carvedilol (Coreg),, pindolol (Visken), and nebivolol (Bystolic). Carvedilol, pindolol, and nebivolol are associated with the least amount of weight gain.

Calcium channel blockers

Most of these medicines are weight neutral, except for verapamil (Calan), which may increase weight slightly. These medicines work by blocking the calcium from going into the blood vessels and heart muscle, which causes relaxation. There are many in this class, but the most common are amlodipine (Norvasc), felodipine (Plendil), nifedipine (Procardia), nicardipine (Cardene), verapamil (Calan), and diltiazem (Cardizem). I use these often depending on the patient's situation.

ACE (angiotensin converting enzyme) inhibitors/ARBs (angiotensin receptor blockers)

These medicines are often the most preferable for treating someone with high blood pressure who doesn't want to gain weight. They work by lowering the activity of the renin-angiotensin-aldosterone system, which basically means you will lower your blood pressure by way of your kidneys, blood vessels, and heart. (I won't bore you with the details.)

The most common ACE inhibitors include lisinopril (Zestril), ramipril (Altace), enalapril (Vasotec), benazepril (Lotensin), and quinapril (Accupril). The common ARBs include losartan (Cozaar), valsartan (Diovan), telmisartan (Micardis), olmesartan (Benicar), candesartan (Atacand), and irbesartan (Avapro). These are generally what I start with, along with lifestyle changes, for blood pressure control.

Diuretics (water pills)

Thiazides are the most commonly used diuretics. Hydrochlorothiazide and chlorthalidone are the most widespread versions. They work by decreasing your blood volume, which will decrease your blood pressure. These are thought to be weight neutral, and I still prescribe them.

There are also other diuretics called loop diuretics. These include furosemide (Lasix), bumetanide (Bumex), and torsemide (Demadex). They aren't used as much for controlling blood pressure but are more frequently used for conditions like heart failure.

Potassium-sparing diuretics include spironolactone (Aldactone) and eplerenone (Inspra). These are generally used for conditions other than high blood pressure (like heart failure or PCOS) but are sometimes used when blood pressure is tough to control.

Others

If your blood pressure is hard to manage, your doctor may prescribe clonidine (Catapres), which changes the effect of adrenaline on your blood vessels. This medicine may also be associated with a little bit of weight gain, like beta-blockers are. While I generally don't like to use this one, sometimes it is necessary.

Dave's Story: Getting Off Blood Pressure Medicine for Good

Dave is a forty-one-year-old truck driver who came to see me for his blood pressure. Technically he didn't meet the obese category for BMI (his BMI was 29, while over 30 is obese). However, his waist was forty-two inches, and over forty inches meets the criteria for "metabolic syndrome." Dave needed a refill of his metoprolol, which he used to control his blood pressure. He said he had gained five or ten pounds since starting the medicine, so before refilling it, I asked if he wanted to make a few lifestyle changes to lose some weight and get off the medicine.

We honed in on some of his nutrition habits. He swapped Gatorade for water while driving (and sometimes Propel, the zero-calorie Gatorade). I also suggested he eat an apple or banana instead of a muffin at his stops. He had a membership at Planet Fitness, so he started on the Planet Fitness plan in this book.

After a couple months, he had lost four inches around his belly and twelve pounds in all. And he no longer needs medication to control his blood pressure. He continues to pump iron and eat better.

Steroids and Hormones

Birth control

There are multiple types of oral birth control that have all been studied for their effects on weight. The one that consistently shows weight gain is medroxyprogesterone acetate (a.k.a., "the Depo shot" or Depo-Provera) and progestin-only oral contraceptives. Combination (estrogen and progesterone) birth-control pills may increase weight in some women.

The copper intrauterine device (Paragard) has no hormonal action and is very effective and weight neutral. There are two levonorgestrel IUDs out there as well (Mirena and Skyla), which haven't been linked to weight gain in studies, although some women report weight gain while using them.

There isn't a lot of data about the weight impact of the vaginal etonogestrel ring (NuvaRing) and arm implant (Nexplanon), but some women appear to gain weight with Nexplanon.

Glucocorticoids

Drugs like prednisone and methylprednisolone are common drugs that can cause significant weight gain. Talk to your doctor about using the lowest dose possible to control your symptoms. Do not stop taking them without talking to your doctor, as this can cause a very serious problem called "adrenal insufficiency."

Hormone Replacement Therapy (Women)

Many women complain of weight gain after menopause. Hormone replacement therapy hasn't been shown to cause weight gain, and it may help with symptoms (such as hot flashes). However, it doesn't cause weight loss. There is some data to suggest that hormone replacement therapy may help to prevent fat from being stored around the belly.

I don't automatically prescribe hormones to women going through menopause, and neither should your doctor. There should be a discussion based on your symptoms and the risks and benefits.

Testosterone (Men)

Testosterone will help with weight loss, but only if you have low testosterone. I do not recommend using testosterone unless you meet the criteria for low testosterone.

Megestrol Acetate (Megace)

This is a progestin drug specifically made for weight gain in those with cancer and other diseases associated with weight loss.

Antihistamines

Taking over-the-counter allergy medicines long term can lead to weight gain. If possible, I would limit their use to short term. These include diphenhydramine (Benadryl), hydroxyzine (Vistaril), loratadine (Claritin), fexofenadine (Allegra), and cetirizine (Zyrtec).

Antiretrovirals/HIV Medicines

I won't go into details about these medications except to point out that they may change the way your body distributes fat (e.g., in the hips or belly).

The Last Word

Finally, it's true that some medicines make it easier to gain weight and more difficult to lose it. You and your doctor should take into account your health, your weight, and your goals when deciding which medication to use. Never start, reduce, or stop taking any kind of medicine without talking to your doctor—he or she is one of the most important members of your support group and can help you reach your weight-loss goals.

9

Frequently Asked Questions about Weight Loss, Diet, Exercise, and Health—and Their Answers

Weight Loss Questions

Why do I always seem to lose weight in spurts?

As nice as it would be for weight loss to happen in a straight line, it almost never works that way. There are many factors that cause your weight to drop erratically, such as retaining or losing water weight.

If you plateau, stick with your plan for at least one or two weeks. If your weight is unchanged after two weeks, you likely need to change your diet and exercise regime.

I gained five pounds over the weekend! How is this possible?

There are many factors that affect your weight besides body fat. The biggest is water. When you eat a large amount of sodium, you'll retain more water and your weight will go up. Eating more food in general can also increase your weight by several pounds.

When you're under stress, your body releases more cortisol, which can also cause water retention. Other hormonal factors can affect how much water you retain, but the bottom line is that it's possible (and normal) to gain several pounds over a few days or even hours. As long as your weight is generally trending downward, don't worry about a short-term weight gain.

When should I think about weight-loss surgery?

When you have a BMI over 40, or a BMI over 35 with another condition like high blood pressure or diabetes and when diet, exercise, sleep, and other lifestyle changes haven't worked for you.

Diet Questions

Do I really need to eat as much protein as you suggest?

Not necessarily, but the goal of the FLP steps is to help you lose little, if any, muscle. Aim to get the recommended amounts to help you retain (and even gain) muscle while losing fat.

Are diet sodas making me gain weight?

No. There is a correlation between drinking diet sodas and weight gain, but that's only because people who are struggling more with their weight tend to drink more diet soda. Carefully controlled experiments have shown that diet sodas can actually be helpful for weight loss. However, your best beverage choice is water. Coffee and unsweetened tea are fine, too.

Don't carbs increase insulin and fat gain?

To make a long story short...no. Calories matter most. Refined carbohydrates like sugar, candy, cereal, and chips can sometimes make you overeat but not because they raise insulin. Basically, highly refined foods can encourage overeating even if you're full. They bypass the normal processes that your body uses to sense when you've had enough to eat.

Whole oats, rice, and legumes are very different from things like candy bars and Pop-Tarts and can be a part of your weight-loss diet. Fruits and vegetables are almost 100 percent carbs and are extremely healthy.

I hate vegetables. Do I have to eat them?

If you're determined not to eat vegetables of any kind, you can stick to fruit and legumes, possibly with some whole grains, to fill out your plate. Before you say you hate vegetables, though, experiment with different types and different ways to cook them—you may find you like some after all.

But I love eating tacos and pizza. How can I give those up?

I love them, too! Try making them at home, where you control how they're made. You'll cut calories and create healthier dishes. You can indulge on a restaurant version once in a while, too.

Vegetables and legumes make feel me gassy and bloated. Should I still eat them?

Maybe. If you feel gassy or bloated, you may not have an adequate variety of gut bacteria to properly digest what you're eating. Eating probiotics and fermented foods may help.

It's also possible that only a few vegetables or legumes are causing problems. Some vegetables tend to be higher in "FODMAPs," or certain kinds of carbohydrates that not everyone is able to digest easily.

You may also just need more time to adapt to your diet and let your gut bacteria catch up with what you're eating.

I heard that there are things in legumes that make them bad for you. Is that true?

Yes, some legumes contain small amounts of certain compounds that *can* be bad for you if you consume them raw. But almost every form of legume you eat is either soaked, canned, or cooked in some way. Other legumes, like peanuts, are perfectly healthy to eat raw. As a whole, legumes are among the healthiest foods you can eat.

Is breakfast really the most important meal of the day?

No. Most data indicates that people who are able to lose weight and keep it off do eat breakfast. But that's not because there's something magical about eating earlier in the day. People who are generally more health conscious are more likely to eat breakfast, possibly because they've been told it's healthy. Some people who lose weight successfully feel that eating breakfast helps them control their hunger. Others delay it or skip it altogether without consequences.

I thought I was supposed to eat six meals a day to increase my metabolism. What's the deal?

Some people believe that if you eat more frequently, you'll increase your metabolism more often throughout the day, and if you don't eat as often, your metabolism will decrease. However, studies have shown that you'll burn the same number of calories eating six meals a day as you do eating two meals per day. In other words, it's your total calorie intake that matters, not how you divide those meals throughout the day.

Isn't meat bad for you?

That depends. Processed meat like hot dogs and salami has been correlated with disease in some studies. You can include lean beef like sirloin and poultry in a diet that is rich in plants, and you can skip meat if you want. Just make sure you're getting enough protein from other sources.

Is saturated fat bad for me?

Saturated fat actually comes in various sizes and forms, so it's hard to say it's bad for you across the board. Refined forms of saturated fat, like butter, should be limited, and other, healthier sources, like olive oil or avocado, should be used instead if possible. I recommend you limit your saturated fat in general. The FLP steps encourage this as well.

Is cholesterol in my food bad for me?

Cholesterol in food doesn't generally affect your blood cholesterol too much. Foods like eggs and shrimp, which are high in cholesterol, can still be a healthy part of your diet.

I don't have a lot of money. How can I eat this food for cheap?
You can eat very cheaply and still get extremely healthy foods. Canned and frozen vegetables are absolutely fine, and frozen fruits, like berries, are awesome and cheap as well. Protein sources like ground turkey, lean beef, and protein powder shouldn't break your bank, and legumes like lentils and beans are inexpensive.

Exercise Questions

Should I do cardio before or after lifting?
Either is fine. I do my cardio after lifting weights.

Should I separate my cardio and lifting sessions?
Don't worry about timing. You can do them together or separately. Do whatever will work for you.

Can I do CrossFit?
Sure! Make sure you find a place that will tailor the program to your needs, though. I also like other small gyms that will assess your movement and skill needs and create a program with you in mind.

I feel like I am always tired and sore. Is it possible to overexercise?
It's best to start out slow and gradually increase your workout volume. If you're so sore that you don't want to or can't exercise, take it back a notch. You may be overtraining. Check in with your support group for advice.

Medical Questions

I thought weight-loss medicines were bad for you. Why would you recommend them?
In the past twenty years, some weight-loss drugs have been taken off the market. However, the medicines we have out now seem to be safe.

My doctor won't prescribe a weight-loss medicine. What should I do?
If you meet the criteria (a BMI over 27 with a weight-related disease, or a BMI over 30), and you really think you need medicine, go to the American Board of Obesity Medicine's website (www.Abom.org) to find an obesity specialist in your area.

My thyroid is normal. However, I read online that I need more testing. Is that true?
There are many claims about the importance of testing thyroid function (e.g., testing reverse T3), but I would be very skeptical of them. The evidence is shaky on the benefits of this kind of testing.

My testosterone is low to normal, and my doctor won't give me testosterone. What should I do?

You can seek a second opinion, but I recommend that you only take supplemental testosterone if you have low testosterone. There are risks involved with taking testosterone if you don't need it.

Can I really still eat carbs even when I am a type 2 diabetic?

Yep! Remember that the best diet is the one that you will stick to long term. If you have prediabetes or type 2 diabetes, you will improve your blood sugar numbers if you eat fewer calories than you burn. Excess fat causes insulin resistance. When you lose weight, the insulin resistance improves. I do like using a lower carb approach—by consuming fewer carbs than normal, you'll lower your blood sugar in the short term, and by losing weight, you'll improve insulin resistance over the long term.

FLP Steps Cheat Sheet

How You Eat:

- Roughly three to four meals per day.
- Mostly plants (vegetables, fruits, legumes) with a serving or two of lean protein at each meal.
- Eat slowly (shoot for twenty minutes).
- Include water, coffee, tea, or other sugar-free beverages. (Protein shakes are an exception.)
- Stop eating before you feel full.
- If you're not losing weight with this meal plan, you may need to track your calories and macronutrients (carbohydrates, fat, protein).

How You Move:

- Shoot for thirty minutes a day of aerobic exercise or "cardio" (equivalent of brisk walking).
- Lift weights two or three days per week.
- Get a pedometer (e.g., Fitbit) and shoot for ten thousand steps daily.
- Stand instead of sitting if possible.
- Get outside and enjoy nature.

How You Live:

- Aim to get seven to eight hours of restful sleep.
- Keep your bedroom environment conducive to sleep.
- If you snore, gasp, or stop breathing at night, get checked for sleep apnea!
- Join an online support group. (Join mine at www.FatLossPrescription.com.)
- Consider hiring a coach if a support group isn't enough. (Check out www.FatLossPrescription.com to learn more about coaching.)
- Develop ways of handling emotions that don't involve food.

Still Not Losing Weight?

- Talk with your doctor about medical issues that could be holding you back and how to address them.
- Talk with your doctor about using a weight-loss medicine. (If your doctor is unable to help with these issues, look for an obesity specialist physician at www.Abom.org.)
- If the FLP steps and other options fail, you may want to consider bariatric surgery. Get a referral to a good surgeon in the area who can help you.

For access to the private Facebook group, other bonuses, and a list references, please go to www.FatLossPrescription.com.

About the Author

D R. SPENCER NADOLSKY is a board certified Family Medicine Physician and a Diplomate of the American Board of Obesity Medicine. His love for lifestyle as medicine began in athletics where he worked hard using exercise and nutrition science to propel himself in football and wrestling. After wrestling at UNC Chapel Hill as the Tar Heel heavyweight and earning a degree in exercise science, he headed to Edward Via College of Osteopathic Medicine in Blacksburg.

During medical school, Dr. Nadolsky attended multiple obesity medicine conferences and realized that he wanted to use the same nutrition and exercise information he learned for athletics but now for the general population and health. After medical school, he attended VCU's Riverside Family Medicine Residency in Newport News to hone his skills. He is currently practicing in Olney, Maryland.

27625986R00070

Made in the USA
Middletown, DE
19 December 2015